Ninjutsu

Spirit of the Unconventional Combat Arts

(Mental Strength and Physical Abilities of the Ninjutsu Masters)

Caridad Barnes

Published By **Caridad Barnes**

Caridad Barnes

All Rights Reserved

Ninjutsu: Spirit of the Unconventional Combat Arts (Mental Strength and Physical Abilities of the Ninjutsu Masters)

ISBN 978-1-77485-443-3

Legal & Disclaimer

The information contained in this book is not designed to replace or take the place of any form of medicine or professional medical advice. The information in this book has been provided for educational and entertainment purposes only.

The information contained in this book has been compiled from sources deemed reliable, and it is accurate to the best of the Author's knowledge; however, the Author cannot guarantee its accuracy and validity and cannot be held liable for any errors or omissions. Changes are periodically made to this book. You must consult your doctor or get professional medical advice before using any of the suggested remedies, techniques, or information in this book.

Upon using the information contained in this book, you agree to hold harmless the Author from and against any damages, costs, and expenses, including any legal fees potentially resulting from the application of any of the information provided by this guide. This disclaimer applies to any damages or injury caused by the use and application, whether directly or indirectly, of any advice or information presented, whether for breach of contract, tort, negligence, personal injury, criminal intent, or under any other cause of action.

You agree to accept all risks of using the information presented inside this book. You need to consult a professional medical practitioner in order to ensure you are both able and healthy enough to participate in this program.

TABLE OF CONTENTS

introduction... 1

Chapter 1: Understanding.................................... 3

Chapter 2: Appearance 8

Chapter 3: Tools.. 16

Chapter 4: Fitness 26

Chapter 5: Ninjutsu Training And Skills.............. 44

Chapter 6: The Occult Pragms And Philosophy Of The Ninja 99

Chapter 7: Warfare Principles And Ninjutsu 134

Chapter 8: Incorporating Ninjutsu Principles For Selfdefense 149

Conclusion 184

Introduction

Welcome. You've already made the first step towards making your life more enjoyable through this book. It might sound like something that you'd like to be saying, but you can be sure that the advice provided in this book isn't being a cliche.

This book will help readers become a ninja in the current world. This isn't just about being physically fit. This is only one part of it. Ninjas introduced a new kind of respect in the world. The mere mention of them could trigger an eerie feeling in even the most obedient of Samurai. They achieved this with an innovative method of thinking. They transformed their environment to gain an advantage by using the use of stealth.

We all believe that it was their fighting abilities that stood out. We shouldn't? We see the ninjas kick people's backs every day on TV. But ninjas weren't famous for their martial arts skills. In fact it's safe to say that Samurai was superior to Ninjas in this area. Ninjas were well-known because of their capability to move and not be noticed. Their greatest strength was that they could move around without being noticed.

This book has been designed to show you all you require to know to be more secure while being living your normal life. It doesn't matter whether you're a broker in the stock market or an athlete, you'll benefit from the knowledge that is provided in this book to gain an advantage. The process of becoming an American Ninja is not about being ripped, quite contrary in reality. It's about preparing yourself to use your environment to your advantage.

Chapter 1: Understanding

The History of the Ninja

There is no way to pinpoint the exact date at which the first ninja appeared from the darkness of history. What we do know is that ninjas were employed to perform the more dangerous tasks that entailed the honor of Samurai. Shinobi (the actual name for the Ninja) is a significant aspect of Japanese folklore. They are believed to descend from an evil demon that was a perfect mix of man and crow. It's more likely that ninjas derived from their very opposite counterparts which were the Samurai in the early period of feudal Japan. Their sly nature makes it almost impossible to pinpoint the exact date.

We do know that the art of Ninjutsu was first to grow around the year 600AD , but prior to the year 907AD. The reason we are able to affirm that ninjas had been present by the year 907 was because this was the year that the art of ninjutsu began to introduced across the continent. The end of the Tang Dynasty plunged China into chaos and forced Chinese commanders to Japan who brought innovative battle tactics and war ideas, which included the art of ninjutsu.

What made the Ninja and Samurai different?

In the beginning, ninjutsu designed to be the force that was opposing to bushido (the code of the Samurai). Samurai believed in honor over everything else, while ninjas were concerned about the success in their task. Also, the ninjas did whatever was necessary to complete their goal. The use of sneak attacks, poisons and even seduction were allowed to the Ninjas, as long as they were able to achieve the accomplishment of their mission.

This is the irony. Samurai lords sometimes were stifled by their own beliefs, so they hired ninjas perform their dirty work to ensure that they kept their hands clear. Ninjas were recruited to serve as assassins, spies, and even planted false information within the ranks of the enemy. Bushido allowed samurais to employ Ninjas to do this without jeopardizing their reputation.

The result was a Samurai's enemies hiring ninjas to serve exactly the same reason. The powerful samurai then encountered a force that scared even the ninjas. Ninjas were a threat that Samurais needed, hated and also feared.

Ninja's Rise and Fall

Ninjas came to their full potential during the turbulent period (1360-1600). The ongoing wars led to the ninjutsu being a necessity for all parties involved.

In the Nanbukucho Wars, ninjas played an important role in the end result: acting as spies on both sides and even helping to destroy south court's Hachiman-vama Fortress. In the end, however, it was only the North Court eventually won the battle.

70 years after that , came an all-out civil war that was known as called the Onin War. Ninjas were prominently featured in this event in the past, even going as far to act as scouts or sneak attackers. They could deter defenders during castle sieges , and provide the army attacking an enormous advantage.

The ninjas, however, had grown so fearful that they might ultimately be targeted by warrior Oda Nobunga. He unified Japan and took over the strongholds of ninjas at Koga as well as Iga. He used massive numbers to bring the ninja to engage in open warfare but this wasn't their forte. Then, he smashed down both strongholds, and scattered the ninja across Kii's mountains. Kii.

Even though their main power bases were destroyed, they remained. Their demise was actually in the Edo Period, which brought peace to Japan. Although their tale may have ended, the ninja's skills and legends will never die.

What can this do for us to be Successful in Today's World?

The ninja emerged from the depths of history with an unorthodox view of life. In a time when the ideals of Bushido were the norm for all combatants, the warriors of the Ninja developed an innovative philosophy that lifted them out of poverty into history. It doesn't mean that you have to begin breaking laws to leave your mark on the history. In fact, it doesn't necessarily mean that the values of the ninja were right. Just learn to look at things from a different perspective and then train yourself to behave in different ways.

The goal is to show how their method of life can be incorporated into the American way of life. In actuality, I can observe some similarities:

A man is dressed in a dark suit. we believe they're successful

Secret service personnel and women are known to dress in dark suits.

We have a saying "nice guys come last" and many people believe in this.

The way we are educated is to look out and outside the boundaries.

The uniforms of the military are designed to are in harmony with the surroundings.

What kinds of things can you see that are reminiscent of an Ninja?

You're not alone, how you dress, the way you carry yourself and even your fitness level ultimately determines your ability to succeed. This book is special. It will teach you how to integrate Ninja-like discipline into your everyday life. You're not going to be taught how to become a spy or assassin. But you will be taught you can become an American Ninja!

Chapter 2: Appearance

What is the best way to Look Like a Ninja

Contrary to popular opinion it's true that appearance is important. There's a saying that says it's what's inside you that counts. I'm not going to argue with this. In fact, I believe it. But, your appearance acts as a mirror which reflects the character of a person. In reality we're all assessed by the appearance of our bodies. Ninja's clothing reveals the inner discipline of a person.

Different types of Ninja Outfits and Accessories

Ninjas did not make their gears solely on appearance. Each piece was utilized for a specific purpose so that no inch of fabric was wasted.

Armor

Ninja armor was Shinobu's most popular kind of attire and, contrary to what is commonly believed it wasn't always black. Ninja's would wear the armor they wore for a variety of different reasons, with the most important being to increase their physical strength over foes. The armor of plates was used in battle to shield against sharp weapons and blunt injuries. In addition, the armor for ninjas was designed to enhance their attack. improved their attack.

Armor can also be customized in a certain extent. While it served some practical use in the past, back when it was at the height of Shinobu's popularity, people who follow the Shinobu code today may be seen wearing mesh armor over their regular attire. It gives them an aura of confidence and confidence.

Cloaks

Cloaks are perhaps the most versatile item of clothing that ninjas can have as they can be used for different reasons. Cloaks can shield you from the elements and be worn during occasions, and serve as a mark of respectability.

Flak Jackets

Flak jackets were utilized to shield the wearer from projectsiles, blunt force trauma and other blunt forces. Additionally, they prevented the possibility of fatal injuries from swords. Flak jackets replaced plate armor during the time of the first Shinobu War.

Forehead Protector

The headband of a ninja was an emblem of their loyalty. It symbolized their achievement as a part of the Shinobu in their village, and also entitled them to enjoy the benefits of this privilege. To be able to obtain their ninja symbol, they was required to be a graduate of the Shinobu of their village.

Full Body Suit

A body suit that is full-length is one piece of clothing that covers your entire body, with the exception of the hands, head and feet of a Ninja. It was designed to be stealthy more than anything else. They are not a problem and may be the most commonly worn ninja outfit available.

Hip Pouch

In general, ninjas carried several hip bags across their back. They were utilized to hold the most basic of items used by ninjas, like shuriken and smoke bombs.

Medical Pouch

As opposed to hip pouches and hip bags they were worn on those buttocks that were worn by the Ninja. They are also bigger for storage of medical equipment for use in the field. Imagine it as an ninja's take on a medical kit for first-aid.

Masks

Masks are among the most renowned attires worn by the Ninjas. However, they weren't always black, as pop culture has conjured in our minds. Ninjas could go to the extent of wearing animal masks. In their prime the mere mention of Shinobu Shinobu caused fear to rooms.

Medical Suit

The medical suit hasn't been very widely used in pop culture, however nevertheless, they were there. Shinobu doctors wore them to distinguish themselves from ordinary Ninjas.

Shuriken Holster

Similar as a hip bag it was designed specifically to hold shuriken or kunai exclusively. It was designed to provide the weapon in a quick and easy manner to use in battle. In most cases the ninjas had to place bandages on the holster to stop it from stopping blood flow.

Straw Hats

The hats were primarily used to hide one's identity. However, they is often seen in Shinobu historical documents. This is understandable for a group which was averse to being shady above all other things.

How to make your Own Ninja Costume

There's a good chance that you're likely to not want to dress as a ninja or unless you're in the desire to make people believe you're breaking into them.. If you're looking to make the most of this, you're likely going to need to wear real ninja gear while practicing. We will however offer few tips to make your everyday clothes more similar to a ninja.

Let's go through the amazing method to make your personal ninja outfit.

Make your Own Ninja Outfit

Although ninja clothing was often dark and sombre, popular culture has led us to think of black as a symbol of ninjas. So, you'll find that you'll benefit the most benefit from creating your ninja costume as dark and as concealed as much. If you reside in a region that is snowy, it is best to go with black over white.

The Headband

What you'll need

1 black T-shirt (big enough to wear)

1.) Place the shirt on an even surface.

2.) Start at the bottom, and fold up until you've got the headband.

3.) The sleeves will create two ends that are easy to tie to each other. They'll likely be visible so we'll protect them by...

A Hood

What will you require

1 black long-sleeved t-shirt

1.) Imagine that you were putting on your shirt, however, stop at your ears, so that your arch is placed between your ears and nose.

2.) 2. Pull your shirt's back to the point that it reaches on top of your head, and over your hair. Then, adjust the shirt so that only your eyeline is visible.

3.) Put the sleeves on your head.

Full Body Suit

What do you need

1 long sleeve, Black T-shirt (loose but not too baggy)

One pair of yoga pants in black (loose but not too baggy)

One pair of athletic black shoes

1.) This is a simple process. It is easy to put on the pants, shirt and shoes as normal. The outfit is intended to be worn for ninja training, so be aware of that. It is unlikely that you would wish to wear this in public unless you wish to attract some very snarky appearances.

Belt

What will you require

1 black t-shirt (larger than the size you wear)

1.) This follows the same concept as the headband except that you wrap it around the waist. The sleeves are tied to your back.

The Easy Way

Naturally, one can shop online for the ninja costume. It's much more of an intellectual method to maintain a ninja mentality rather than to present yourself as a ninja other people. Remember, ninjas utilized their clothes for a variety of reasons however none was just to look cool. Their clothes helped them remain in the dark, frightened and also provided the tools needed for their tasks.

Ninja Tips that can be incorporated into with a Lifestyle that's Everyday

The world is a task, so here are some daily techniques that can give you the same advantages as a ninja, while also appealing to the popular society in American life.

Tip 1 Dress to impress

It's always been proven that people who dress in the way they want to will be more successful. If you're using the ninja mentality to enhance your lifestyle, then the it is likely that you would not wish to appear like the typical burglar. There are ways you can bring the ninja approach to American lifestyle to enhance your life.

Wear clothes that match your surroundings. Here are a few examples:

If it's snowing outside, try wearing white clothing for the day.

Wear dark clothing to formal events at night.

Dress in suits that complement the office setting. For instance, if your office is white, then wearing a dark suit will make a stark contrast. But, you should only apply this to jobs that permits it. If not, you are able to wear ninja clothes under your regular work attire.

Tip 2. Remain Secretive

Ninjas are skilled at the art of stealth first and foremost. It's not as if you can hide in every corner or launching out of the ceiling to make a grand entrance (how awesome would that be!). In reality, you must have stealth included in everyday routine to keep the ninja lifestyle.

Learn to walk with a calm and steady pace. It begins with choosing the right footwear and can extend to walking "toes initially". When you first walk on your heels, it produces a thud which will cause you to be in surprise. Don't be one of the people whose footsteps are heard from across the room.

Controlling your breathing is a second technique that you can employ in every day life. Additionally, it's healthier and will boost your energy levels. There are three kinds of breathing: normal, exercise and scared. Find out how to manage each.

Don't share information for free. Talking about water bottles and gossip is a rite of passage that is common in our modern world. It's not a good habit for anyone adopting the style of an Ninja. When speaking to colleagues or acquaintances, don't divulge too many details. Be discrete or you could be shocked.

Select a stylish pair of shoes for your everyday use. If you're in your home, you can try wearing just socks. Do not wear shoes in leaf- or grassy places. You can use flexible soles for tasks like normal walking, and other things that require you to walk in public. I'm sure you've got the concept. Select shoes that are as silent as you can.

Chapter 3: Tools

A Ninja's Equipment

In addition to their clothes Ninjas also had specific equipment they had to utilize to make it through dangerous missions. If you're thinking of becoming an American Ninja, then chances are that you'll need to learn at the very least the basics of how to use the weapons.

The Ninjato

The ninjato was also known by the name of shinobigatan or the ninjaken, the Ninjato was the most powerful weapon. They were shorter than other swords of the time. They were designed solely for ease of use. In the end Ninjas might have struggled with the ability to stealth if they had the bulky sword around their back.

The absence of any historical evidence is a challenge to establish the precise use of the ninjato and we have to speculate. The visual and literary media tend to portray the ninja using the same technique as masters of katana, while other media illustrate them using the reverse gripping technique.

Safety Alert

Keep in mind that any sword is a dangerous weapon. It is not recommended to use an actual sword for your own personal training. You can substitute it with a homemade and secure replica. A wooden sword can be an excellent substitute.

Learn to Make a Homemade Ninjato

Here's how you can create an uninvolved replica of the Ninjato.

What will you require

1 bit of PVC pipe, about three hand lengths. (Grip)

1 flat piece wooden material (about 1"by 1"). Its length must be approximately three times the length of your handle (Blade)

1 square piece of tin

One roll of electrical tape

1.) Apply tape to the PVC pipe onto the wood piece that is flat. Continue to tape all the way up to the handle until you've completely covered the pipe with PVC while attaching the blade. Try repeatedly swinging the handle to ensure that the blade stays in place against the handle.

2.) Then, cut the tin square through the blade before sliding it over the handle. Make sure you place enough tape beneath it to hold the tin to the handle.

3.) Find a space that is open and swing the sword like when you were practicing. If the sword is able to stand through a full session, then it is likely to be fine.

Shuriken

Also known as ninja stars or throwing stars. The shuriken has become the most popular weapon used by ninjas in popular culture. They are mostly used to throw and are an additional weapon for both samurai and ninja.

What is the best way to Make a Paper Ninja Star

It's recommended to be able to have a flat surface, such as the table or desk that you can fold up.

1.) Start with a standard sheet of sheet of paper (8.5 11.5" x 11"). Place it flat on the floor and create an angle fold in such a way that the sides and top of the paper meet. This creates a huge right-angled triangle that has an extended bottom. Flip the paper over and fold the bottom upwards to make sure it is in line with the other triangle. This will make a visible fold in the area where you folded it.

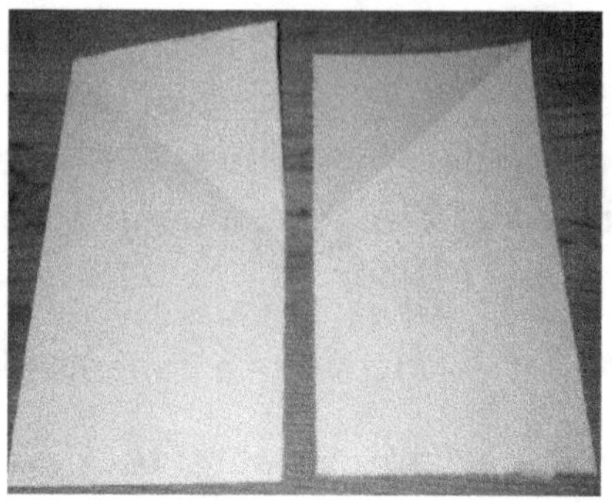

2.) Cut the last crease until you have an uncut square of paper. Cut that square in half, so that you're left with two pieces of paper.

3.) Then, take the two halves, cut them into half, and put them in a position where the open ends face one another. Then fold the tops in such a way that when they are placed together, they make an arch. Then fold the bottoms opposite directions. This will create what appears to be the child's version of a rocket ship.

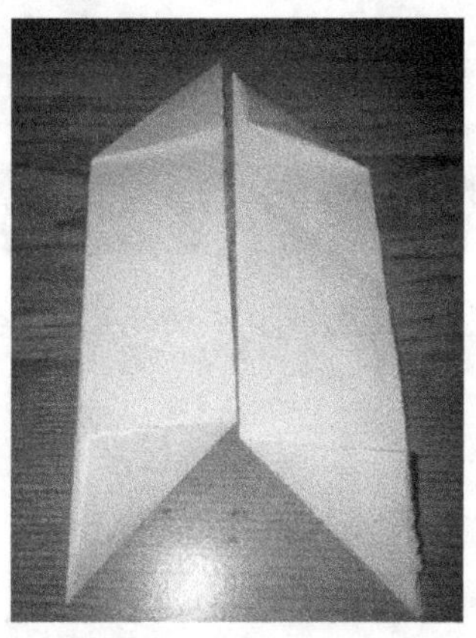

4.) Here is the time to get difficult. Begin by creating an arc by folding the part of the body so that it's aligned with the bottom and top of your "kid's rocketship."

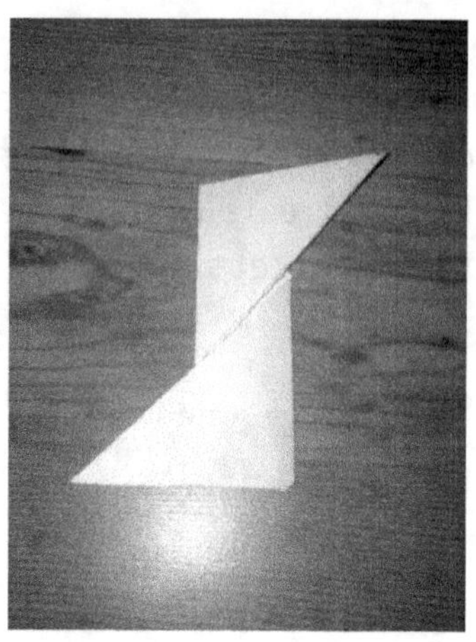

5.) Repeat the step before with the second half.

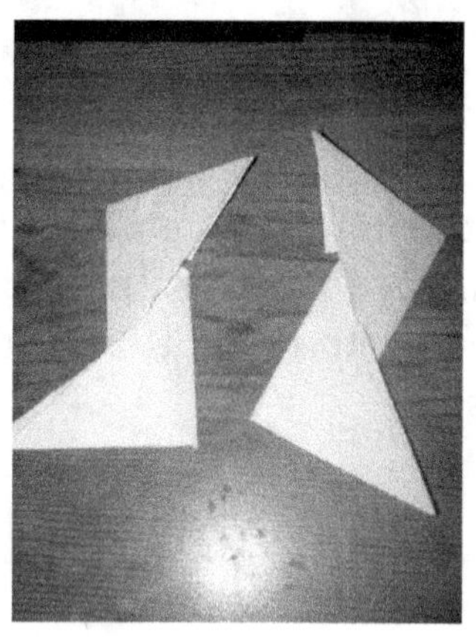

6.) Put both halves together to ensure that the openings face to one side. This part is difficult so take the image below for a guideline.

.

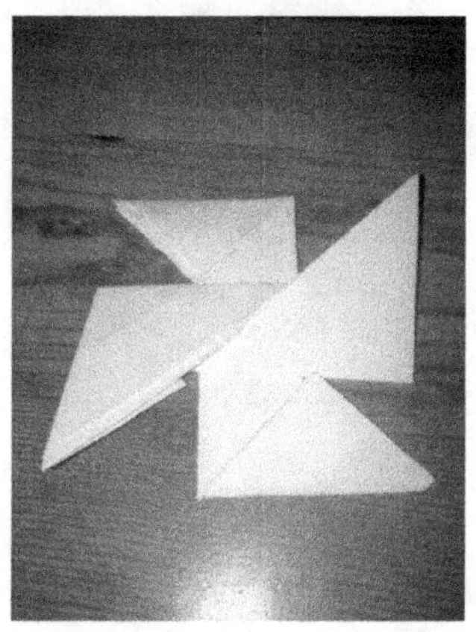

7.) Lastly fold the part of the star to create an opening on the opposite piece. Repeat the process on the other piece, then turn the entire thing on its side and continue.

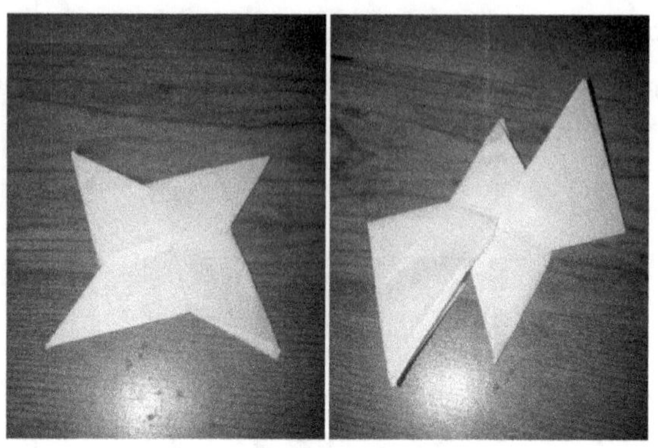

Congratulations. Now you're a Ninja star!

Nun chucks

Nun chucks weren't an everyday weapon for the Ninja, but they were utilized in certain situations. Ninjas trained to use them in those rare occasions.

How to make Paper Nunchucks

Always, safety must be the main concern when learning to be Ninja. Therefore, paper nun chucks are the best option. They are extremely simple to make.

What will you require

2 pieces of paper

2 papers

Duct tape

Strings that are braided or roped

Begin by rolling the paper piece by piece and apply duct tape to hold it in the desired position. You will end up with two Cylinders.

Attach the end of the rope/string onto the cylinder. Wrap the cylinder with a newspaper and then tape it shut. What you have is a more substantial cylinder, with the rope or string attached to it. You can probably see where we're going by this.

Repeat the same procedure using the second cylindrical.

Use the nun chucks to swing them and check to see if they can stand up to the strain. If they do, you've got a safer option to practice with.

Chapter 4: Fitness

Ninja Training

Now you have a better idea of the ninja's traits. You may even have the gear you need (hopefully you've opted to use only safe wooden and paper-based weapons). You'll be amazed at how much you're on the right track. Knowing what makes a ninja such a powerful weapon is one thing. Getting in shape physically is another. This is the reason this part of the game comes into play.

Do you believe that ninjas become experts in the blink of an eye? Sure, but it took many hours of intense physical and mental training. While I'm not saying you'll have to put in endless hours in training. In reality, just one hour per day could equip you for the challenges of the world of today in a way which seems like a stretch in the moment.

A Ninja Lives in Zen

The very first activities you should begin your path to becoming an ninja are not involving exerting your body physically. Your mental strength is just as crucial. In the end an ninja will always be serene and composed. They don't allow their emotions to take over while on a mission. They remain in a state of mind that is known as

Zen. The ability to be cool as the ninja requires many hours of training.

Breathing

Above all else, stay relaxed. Relax and take deep breaths every time you experience strong emotions.

Do not be worried about what other people have to say about You

Learn to let go of the things that other people have said about you, whether positive or negative. You are in no way in control of over what other people think, so avoid dwelling on it. Never argue with someone who's talking negatively about you.

Learn to Respect

I think respect may be among the most misunderstood skills in the present day. There are people who have no idea of respect, while other believe that people should be respectful by bowing down to their every desire. Always show respect to all people, including yourself. A little bit of respect can go far.

Keep your eyes on the important Things

Being stressed over small events puts your feelings to tip over. They become more difficult to control , and it's easy to cause you to fall over. If you can learn to not be distracted by the little things, then you'll be more motivated to remain in control even when confronted with greater challenges.

Do not show emotion.

A ninja isn't one to display emotions that can be dangerous to their own safety. It doesn't mean you aren't feeling these emotions, after all humans are human beings and are not able to prevent our emotions from arising. However, allowing others to view these emotions exposes weaknesses that can be exploited by many.

Learn to Turn Off your Inner Ninja

If you don't want to become a machine that is unable to enjoy a laugh then you must discover how to silence your inner Ninja. The general rule is to utilize your ninja skills when wear the right clothes. Consider this for a second. The real ninja warriors were spies that were required to hide their identities. Do you think they were out and about in a day-to-day manner without emotions? They'd be a noticeable sight and not been quite Ninja-like.

What exactly is Parkour?

Parkour enthusiasts seek to maneuver through the world as swiftly as they can. It's a great method of get fit and have lots of enjoyment. If you're training to become an American Ninja, it's an excellent way to master how to stealth. Parkour will force you to look at the world in a different way. Instead of following the plan laid out before you by a certain architect, your brain will begin to look for other methods of getting from A to B.

Parkour began with France as a tactic for military use. training method to improve the soldier's tactical skills.

What is the reason people do parkour?

The first thing to note is that it's entertaining. People are able to literally make their environment an enormous playground. In reality, lots people have admitted to pretending to be the ninja in their parkour practice. Why is that? A ninja must be an expert in their surroundings. This is the reason why it's included throughout the book.

Parkour is an excellent exercise option because it involves running and swinging, climbing, leaping, and occasionally crawling. It's not just great exercise for the body, but also an excellent exercise for the mind.

Parkour challenges an individual's physical and mental acuity. As time passes, parkour can dramatically increase the strength of an individual and coordination. They are also two crucial skills needed by an professional ninja.

Parkour helps prepare you for extreme situations. Parkour offers the ability and physical endurance to be able to survive in the event of a dangerous situation to occur. Consider it this way. If you were in the threat of death Do you have the skills to survive and escape? This is perhaps one of the main reasons to develop your Ninja skills.

Additionally, it teaches the ability to think creatively. It forces people to be open to the world around them and to learn to engage with things in the most productive ways that are possible. In fact, I'd even claim that parkour could spill into other areas of your life, making every day more fun and creative.

What can this do to help you become an even better Ninja?

Parkour wasn't mentioned since it's an element of your ninja-training. It's there because I believe that knowing this line of thought is essential for enhancing your mental capabilities.

Ninjas' mental strength was their greatest weapon. Their ability to think outside of the box helped them succeed when other people failed. If there's a wisdom to be gained from this experience Let it be that in the future you will not look at your surroundings in the same way architects would like you to consider it. The day is here when that you awake from your daydream that the majority of people fall victim to. They simply follow the general flow , and when something unexpected occurs, they are a victim of panic. most dangerous adversary. This is not going to occur to you. You'll become the next American Ninja.

Ninja Training Exercises

Ninjas possess three fundamental skills that need to be taught:

- Bodyweight Strength

- Endurance

Agility

Therefore, we'll base our exercise program around these three capabilities. Let's begin with strength.

Bodyweight Strength

Let's get this straight. The strength of all the muscles does not matter for Ninjas. They just require the strength needed to carry their body. This is called bodyweight strength. Any strength exercise you engage in should comprise exercises that use your body weight, such as pull-ups, push-ups and any other exercise that utilizes your body weight to provide resistance.

Feel free to develop your own bodyweight exercise program.

This is a fantastic bodyweight strength set to help you get to the right place. The set of exercises will strengthen your upper and lower bodies and everything else between. Because it relies on your body weight to create resistance, it will assist to build strength and endurance through your body weight.

Exercise Instructions

The aim is to go through this whole list of exercises without stopping. Make use of your own judgement to determine when you should stop for a rest before you begin.

1. 5 pull-ups (with towel) Instead of taking grip on the bar put a towel over it and hold the bar at each end. Use it to do the pull-ups. This will help improve your grip.

2. Fist Pushups 20: Perform twenty push-ups . Instead of using your palms as hands utilize your fists instead to help support your body's weight.

3. Hindu Pushups x 20: Hindu pushups are a excellent addition to any workout routine. Here's how to do them. Start in the typical pose of the pushup however, with your elbows raised and your legs further and farther apart from your hands. The goal is to form the shape of a V. In a

swooping motion then lower your body to allow your hips to drop closer to the floor, while your chest and head are moving upwards. As you descend, move fluidly. When you climb, you should swing forward until the point at which the end of your motion arcs your back, and your eyes look up at towards the ceiling. In the end, return to the place from which you began.

Hindu pushups require a bit but of time to master them.

4. V-Ups x 10: Lay on your back, and then spread your arms across your head. Then, lift your legs and arms to each other.

5. Knees-to Chest x10: Sit down and stretch your legs. Lean slightly back, then raise your legs, bent and making them closer in your chest possible.

6. Pendulum Leg Lifts 10 Place your feet in a flat position on your back, and hold your legs straight in the air, while keeping your knees in place. Drop your feet down to the left and then back to the center, then to the right, then back to the center.

After you've completed these exercises, take a brief time to rest, and then do them again in the number of times you feel is needed. The goal is to complete this exercise for at least 20 minutes without a break. It will take some time to get to this point in your training.

Endurance

The strength of your body isn't enough. If you're looking to become Ninja, then you have to increase strength to maximum levels you can.

In our modern society it's quite easy to get lazy. There are buses that will go wherever we'd like to go, vehicles that are affordable for the majority of family members, and benches on every corner. Ninjas didn't have these amenities and consequently they weren't faced with the same temptations we are. This means that you'll be much more difficult in improving your endurance than past Ninjas.

In the end, the best way to build for endurance and speed is running. If Americans would start taking short walks instead of using buses for a mile, we wouldn't be suffering from obesity. So, starting now, you must begin thinking like an Ninja. If possible you can walk or work to the place of your choice.

If you're employed for just a few miles away from your home, you can you should jog every morning to work in the event of rain.

If you're working within a reasonable distance , but too far to run, buy a bike and take it to work.

A simple change to your lifestyle will build your endurance and make you feel fantastic (once you've passed the initial fatigue phase). Do not think about your morning coffee. Running in the morning will bring you such energy you'll be amazed at what you did before.

Agility

We are now moving on to advanced ninja-training. The exercises for agility can also improve your endurance. That's the reason we have mentioned daily endurance improvements rather than workouts. You'll need think outside the box to learn the fundamentals of agility. This is where an elementary knowledge of parkour will come into play. Here are a few options:

Playgrounds

Playgrounds are an excellent spot to try parkour. They are equipped with everything we require to improve our agility. Additionally, if you have children, then playing in playing in the park is a wonderful option to spend time with them. It's a healthier alternative to watching television or video games.

Here are a few items found in playgrounds which can help you improve your agility:

Monkey Bars Monkey bars are an excellent way to practice some of the parkour techniques discussed previously in the chapter. This includes climbing, swinging, leaping, and even landing.

Balance Bar: Many of playgrounds are equipped with the balance bar. If they don't, they are more likely to feature railings which could serve the same purpose.

It is possible to search the internet and look for parksour-themed playgrounds within your region. If they are, then that's excellent! If not, you'll need to settle for whatever you have on hand.

What is the best way to locate a Quality Training Location

It is likely be the toughest part of your ninja-training this is the reason I've dedicated an entire section of time to finding an ideal location to improve your agility. Each location is different, and this should be a judgement that you make. Here are the traits you should be looking for.

Obstacles

We're trying to find obstacles that will hinder our training of all of the agility techniques that we discussed earlier. This includes:

Dropping and jumping

- Balancing

Cat Climbs

Vaulting

The best place to train is one that has various objects of different in height. This way you can practice vaulting on different levels. The walls that are high should be beyond reach, but not overly high. The areas you jump in should be safe , so that should you fall, you do not hurt yourself.

Safety

Once again, I'll emphasize the importance of being safe. Check that the objects you use fall apart when they are used. Broken glass, rusty, exposed nails are another issue. In addition, dirt and grass grounds are better than asphalt and concrete.

Legal

Make sure you're not intruding onto private property. Certain properties will have clearly visible indications that your you are not allowed to do so. This is strictly to safeguard the owner from legal consequences. Always adhere to the local laws.

Large Area

The bigger the area for practice then the better. Greater areas offer greater flexibility and space to train. Try to find area that meets all the previous requirements, and is also big enough.

Skills that parkour/playgrounds should train

Balancing

Balancing is one of the most important skills for Ninjas. Find something that will help you improve your coordination and balance when you're doing your everyday workouts. It can be as simple as being able to stand on one leg, but when you find the obstacle courses, make sure to find a deck to walk along.

Walking and running

Naturally, you'll need to increase your stamina, which is why running can be the most effective method of doing this. It's easy to find a place to run. Walking to work each day is an excellent method to boost your endurance. But, running to work can increase your endurance.

As you're preparing to become a ninja you'll also need to improve your stealth. Learn to run and walk as quiet as you can with the help of landing onto your foot and then gently sliding into your heel with every step.

Dropping and jumping

Jumping is among the abilities that parkour is well-equipped to train. Similar is the case of falling. Training for these skills should be done whenever you can. In addition, you need to master them without a fuss.

The act of jumping and dropping is as easy as jumping down a flight of steps or as complicated like climbing up a tree then dropping it down.

In addition, when first practicing your drop technique make sure you only drop from places that are not more than 5 feet tall. Dropping too high of an area can lead to injury.

Tic-Tac

A Tic-tac is an impromptu wall-climb as well as an incline. It lets you climb places higher than by jumping normally. You've likely seen this technique on TV where a person makes use of the wall to get rid of to get to the top of the hill. In the event that two walls lie located close in proximity, this could be repeated to access an area that is otherwise unaccessible. Don't attempt to play tic-tac over unsafe distances.

Landing

Knowing how to safely land is among the most crucial elements of being a Ninja. A successful landing must provide three crucial elements:

1. Should not cause any discomfort.

2. It is best to be silent.

3. Allow yourself to be able to instantly be able to immediately get up.

Utilizing a railing, you can work on balance and landing simultaneously. Then, you can walk along the railing. at the point you are close to the finish, leap off and take off and land.

Two-Foot Landing

Always opt for a landing with two feet instead of a one-foot landing. A landing that is one foot long is more difficult to control and creates more stress to your body. Furthermore, there is no option to soften the landing. It is crucial to land gently for staying hidden.

To ensure as smooth and smooth a landing you can you should bend your knees when you fall (make sure you don't extend your knees more that 90 degrees). If you're jumping at an angle that is forward let your body receding and then utilize your hands to take the force. It is important to begin training starting at lower levels and gradually increase your height.

Rolling

This is a must in order to stay safe when jumping from higher places. Additionally, it slows (quiets) landings at higher heights and allows Ninjas to make use of their momentum to react quickly upon landing.

Although it's a great ability to acquire but it's not a necessity since you shouldn't jump from such a high point. It can be risky for those who aren't properly trained physically and mentally.

Learn to roll in emergency situations only. Don't be a ninja who jumps from high places a regular part of your ninja's training.

Vaulting

Vaulting is employing your hands and arms to move an object to remove it. It's a crucial ability for the Ninja. In the end, you aren't going to want to be being slowed down because you fail to make a leap that's only a couple of feet too high. It wouldn't be very ninjalike of you. These are the most common forms of vaulting that they need to be taught:

1. Security Vaults: This method is the one that sets the other up and is typically performed as you slowly approach an obstruction. It is where beginners need to begin.

2. Speed Vault The Speed Vault is exactly the identical to the security vault, with only one difference: it's performed while running.

3. Lazy vault: The type of vault is ideal for those who approach at an angle. If your body is advancing over an obstacle and making use of one arm for pushing it over it, you're doing the lazy vault. It is likely that you have performed this at least once throughout your lifetime.

4. Kong Vault: Its name comes in Planet of the Apes. Apes are often seen Kong Vaulting over police vehicles. This is a technique that is advanced that should be only attempted by people with sufficient expertise.

5. Dash Vault: This is identical to The King Vault but instead of jumping first with your feet it is a leap of the head first. The Dash vault is one of the more advanced, and is only for people with many years of vaulting experience.

Climbing

Climbing is a crucial skill for an professional ninja (seems they possess a variety of valuable abilities). While training, avoid climbing dangerous distances. The general rule is to never go higher than you're willing to jump.

As it's difficult to locate suitable areas to climb in real life however, there are a few great alternatives. Choose a bar for pull-ups, but instead of gripping the bar, you can wrap an object with a towel and then hold it while lifting yourself up. This will use the same muscles as pull-ups , but will also improve your grip.

Wall Run

A successful wall race includes a person running through, jumping, climbing and hanging in one move. This allows you to climb a steep wall at an extremely rapid rate. This should not be attempted by anyone who is new to climbing however. Even the most experienced athletes have problems when it comes to wall run.

Cat Leap

This is a mix of both a climb as well as a jump. Cat leaps are typically utilized to bridge gaps when the landing point needs the user to swing and hang off the target instead of landing. The reason is clear The wall or landing spot is too high for you to stand in your shoes. Therefore, you make a swing toward the landing spot then hang on and then lift yourself up.

Swinging

Swinging is pretty easy to explain. It helps improve grip strength and the ability to move.

Chapter 5: Ninjutsu Training And Skills

With regard to their role and their role, it is clear that the ninja of the past were very adept at the capabilities of the body and mind. The methods for training that believe to have employed to bring to fruition a powerful body and sharp sense were such thatat the end of the training the ninja would be able to accomplish amazing physical feats.

Here are just a few examples.

It is believed that a ninja could cover more than 70 miles on foot without a hint of fatigue, in just one day.1 He was used to surviving for long periods of time without proper nutrition, and was able to go without food or even sleeping for a couple of days, without complaint.2,3 Actually The Gunpo Jiyoshu and other texts provide this information in a clear manner by describing the recipes for "hunger pills" that could to sustain a shinobi during an extended mission.

The feats appear to be, on the surface out of the realms that are to be "natural" human capability that require a certain level of sedulity during training, a fact that could be one of the factors that contribute to the myths that surround the supernatural abilities of a shinobi. When you examine the shinobi's image, it becomes apparent that these were just humans who flexed their determination to achieve goals through any means that were available to them by their human nature. Also, the feats they accomplished can be replicated by anyone who has the right attitude with a healthy physique, sharp mind, and a successful training technique.

The skills emphasised in the family lineage Ninjas were, typically speaking, well trained, light-operative (though it was definitely not an everyday). The body's composition gave them the ability to use certain actions that the average person would find to be a bit unconventional and difficult. For instance, in the case that the mission was to be completed in a way that required the absence of any trace of his movements an ninja may require making use of his upper body strength and stability to stick to rafters and rooftops.4 Shinobi-Hiden talks of the use of the kunai (a trowel like digging device) to climb over fortifications, as well as attaching to exterior surfaces of structures. In addition, based on the conditions, he was agile enough to climb over various kinds of walls and fences to ensure that there were no visible tracks on ground below.5

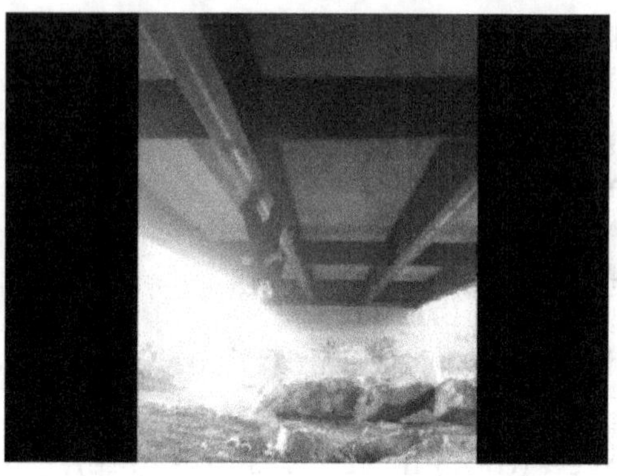

These were not the only way that shinobi were able to disguise their movements, however. There were other methods, such as making prints that appeared to were part of a mysterious or famous creature, or moving sideways, using a method known as Yoko-Aruki. This was done in order to confuse enemies in the direction that the Shinobi was traveling.6

The essence of Ninjutsu

The curricula are established and technical

information that determines the nature of ninjutsu's power isn't

In the near future, it is imperative to attempt to understand

the nature of ninjutsu.

Zhoughari believes that this is because of Ninjutsu's core is

is protected by the inexorably esoteric property is protected by inexorably esoteric properties, the student

In order to find it, you'll need to be involved in processes of

"initiation" as well as spiritual improvement prior to the attainment of any

The depth of understanding that communicates the core of art.9 This refinement of the spirit was believed to be approached

by a shinobi to be an important and beneficial exercise by a shinobi as a necessary and worthwhile activity

the realities of war always called one to think about

their mortal state,10 resulting in the connection between ninjutsu and death.

to specific religious practices to certain religious practices, such as Shugendo and

Shingon Buddhism.

Without this type of spiritual initiation Zoughari

The author asserts that it is impossible to comprehend the core of

Ninjutsu can be considered a martial art even from an intellectual point of view. But,

Unflinchingly, we can still attempt to uncover the

The essence of the matter is revealed by using the tools of logic.

The most interesting thing to observe about this subject is that there's a single

could draw a conclusion about the fundamentals of ninjutsu

through reading from 'Seishin' (correctness of mind) in the

Bansenshukai and understanding the reason for the chapters

The details of it were also included in the text.

Fortunately, Fujibayashi expounds on their

importance.

He states that in the light of the possibility

Utilization of applications for ill and technical know-how

in contained in Bansenshukai included in the Bansenshukai. It was crucial that the concept of a right mind be

The text is communicated to the reader in such a way that they can prevent the creation of criminals. The author explains that, without this notion of a 'correct mind the text could be viewed as an information source to any criminal looking for strategies to

serving self-interested and evil motives.

Based on this, one can easily conclude that

The ninjutsu heart does not include the skills or

methods, for instance, when this is the case one could

Simply emulate a method of ninjutsu, and then call yourself a

shinobi. But no, Fujibayashi. Fujibayashi. The essence of ninjutsu was in

the motivations and beliefs that the individual practitioner (see chapter

3).

If these chapters on "Seishin' are not filled with the

an essential ingredient in ninjutsu then why

Fujibayashi consider it necessary to include them to

How can you distinguish ninjutsu from criminality? The reason

insists that Seishin is essential to understand

ninjutsu.

In addition"Shochi II" from Fujibayashi's book

The following outline the fundamental qualities of a 'jonin' or master.

Shinobi who is believed to possess a sense of essence

of the of the (note that the term "art" of the art does not mean of a social

hierarchy). These are the characteristics:

1. He must appear "gentle" and upright

2. Maintain a healthy and fit body

3. Communicate fluently and have a an unbreakable mind that is indestructible to fraud

4. Be aware about Confucianism and Buddhism

5. Be careful not to get caught up in arguments. be known as a trustworthy person

6. It is essential to be aware of different cultures and geographical regions.

7. You should be proficient in the process of writing, creating strategies, as well as all the other ninjutsu-related skills (those defined by the Bansenshukai, both implicit and explicit)

8. Perform well as a dancer, musician and impersonator11

The Kiai

Many who have seen films about martial arts are

is associated with familiar with "spirit sound" or"kiai" that is often used

to interfere with an enemy's concentration or focus.

The actor in the lead role in these films emits a

A powerful and abrupt "YAHH! !" just prior to hitting the

The opponent is hit hard with a powerful punch. The scream of the opponent is one such

In fact, it's almost as if an energy force existed.

activation to channel through the hero's

body to build endurance.

It's the way it is in movies too however, what exactly is it?

Concerning real-time fighting? Do kiais that are robust result in

tangible results against an enemy in a real war? Did you experience

Shinobi are trained in any method that has anything to do with the Kiai?

Gingetsu Itoh could have something to offer in answer to this type of question. According to Itoh the method of protection employed by

Shinobis that were used for the capture of the opponent's

focus or breaking an focus of the opponent is known as Shun.

Kan Sa-Yo12.

In discussing the application of the technique,

Itoh explains that it operates through the use of an

an inborn instinct to "wince" in the body to "wince" or "blink".13 In this short

interval, the shinobi , whose actions caused such reflexes.

is quick to flee in a bid to disappear away from the view of the

confused opponent.14 The goal is to instantly react

to the appearance of the enemy Shun to the presence of the enemy with Kan SaYo in the presence of the enemy with Shun Kan SaYo

The enemy is able to react with violence. This is the strategy however, how does it get done? What is the procedure?

can be used to facilitate to achieve the response you want?

Itoh states that one must shout "like the sound of a lion"15 and offers a chance for theories that the Shinobi could not have just found a use by using the kiai however, if scientific evidence is true In Itoh's account of Shun Ka SaYo further supports the notion that the Ninja were soldiers who witnessed human behavior during war and analyzed the behaviors that they could take advantage of. How did they do it?

An extremely lucid book that focuses on the psychological effects of fighting and killing. in to offer assistance The book is titled On Killing written by Lieutenant. Colonel. Dave Grossman.

Grossman describes that intra-species aggression, like that which occurs in war is observed to disrupt the concept of fight or flight in our psychological responses to stress.

Contrary to inter-species violence (against nonhumans) in which the actions are a reflection of this model, intra-species aggression is a part of the fight-or-flight strategy to "include posture and submission".16

Posturing is a standard method used by many species to respond to threats within species to signal power and dominance. It is rare that the actions in these circumstances escalate into a full-on fight to the end with one of the members belonging to the same species. In this way this phenomenon could be viewed as an attempt by evolutionarily adaptive species to maintain a social order in which everyone is dependent one another in some way. In lieu of killing a helpful member of the species one is a part of in an intraspecies conflict are more likely to subdue or flee from the dominant animal, and thus maintain the status of a lesser social animal, and in fact, this trend is observed in humans.

According to Rory Miller in his publication Meditations on Human beings are involved in an interspecies form of aggression that is used to determine of social standing. It is referred to as "the Monkey Dance", Miller clarifies that posture is a part of displaying dominance , which can degrade into an aggressive behaviour that does not usually cause death.17 In these situations If one's posture or presence is adequate, any contest to status could be avoided completely. What does this have to do with Kiai?

With these understandings of human and animal psychology Kiais can be considered to be an element of human behavior in situations where an interspecies conflict is amplified.

An excellent illustration of this comes in the form of a story about Toshitsugu Takamatsu, the renown instructor in Maasaki Hatsumi. The story is set in the classroom of Takamatsu's sensei Toda. A student from a different school was there to test the methods taught by Toda's school. In the tradition, Takamatsu was believed to be high-ranking, would be the perfect candidate to face the rival. However, unexpectedly, a pupil with lower rank, a lack of fighting skills and a fervent desire to uphold the name at the university, walked up to the challenger in a loud screaming and began to move towards him. The outcome was that the challenger was forced to submit without a fight with the lower student. Why? because of the expressions of dominance and power which were followed by an "demonic" face.18 This was the "posturing" of the child that scared the opponent enough to prompt an submission.19

It is important to consider that in regard to past battle, Grossman explains that posturing and screams, in particular screaming, was an important factor in winning during the course of battle.20

What can we conclude from this? In the first place, when we consider that the sources used by Itoh are reliable We can see evidence that the shinobi of the past were in fact warriors and had created techniques that capitalized on emotional responses to inter-species aggression. Furthermore using the kiai technique by shinobi in escape or fighting is historically proven.

the Human Brain and the Human Mind

The abilities of observation Shinobi had

might have played a role in terms of understanding someone's

the mind via non-verbal signals. Even though it is today regarded as to be a

Superstitious and flawed Shinobis of the past were flawed and had superstitious capabilities.

You will find a lot of value in the process of the person's

physical and behavioral characteristics to be included physical and behavioral characteristics to include it

their manuals, and the Shoninki.21 There is a lot of what they wrote is

It was said that "physiognomy" from Natori Masatake.

It could be that it is only a figment of imagination. But,

if you think about what else has been to be written in regards to a inquiring about what else is written about a

observational skills and their knowledge of culture

Human psychology and custom human psychology, it is reasonable to say

that the ninjas were, in a certain degree that they were able to read

individual's mind. How?

Natori Masatake says the reading of the human

The mind is a difficult task to accomplish. A shinobi operating in this

ability must be able to evaluate the mindset of a person

Without the person being aware of it and must also be able to master

the ability of kiruma ni Kakuru, which is the knowledge of

the mind of another and the acquisition of knowledge through

flattery.22

It is easy to see the practical benefits of using

To gain information, flattery is a common tactic. Rarely does anyone want to.

Be complimented by showing affection with gestures

Commentaries that inflate their self-worth

The target might be hidden from view, but it is possible to reach it.

Enjoy the presence of the Shinobi. The Shinobi are so popular that they have even become a part of the shinobi's daily life.

Shinobi might subtly ask questions about when they are not there.

Answers are designed to address specific areas of concern.

Informational interest. The target might become so used to the shinobi's presence, that he/she might carelessly reveal mission-relevant information. Combine this with the ability to interpret non-verbal body language accurately and you have a form mind reading.

Modern research supports this claim by showing that most human communication and intent is non-verbal. Some estimates suggest as high as 60%. This observation is also a practical consequence of this observation. Criminal investigators often use non-verbal cues to determine if a suspect's story can be believed. Members of the United States have consistently recognized that non-verbal gestures can indicate malicious intent.

Secret Service.23

However, despite all of the above, there are still

Skeptics who are still skeptical about the reliability of using

Non-verbal behavior analysis is a way to see inside the mind.

Concerning those who find the claim that nonverbal behavior reliability is unpalatable.

Non-verbal reading can be marked as superstitious (it is possible).

It is utterly pointless and informative to mention that modern technology is

This practice is still relevant and applicable today.

Terry v. Ohio, a Supreme Court decision

1968 This decision allows law officers to

Stop and frisk people without a warrant

They have sensed non-verbal clues that criminal intent was being expressed.

This is why non-verbal reading is so reliable and effective.

has been established in a legal domain together with the

Understanding that it can be a transferable skill.

Legal ramifications in the context of contemporary

society.24

How to Infiltrate A Castle

There are many ways you can sneak into a castle depending on your circumstances. The Koka and Iga manuals provide a list of some that is worth noting along with information on how to gauge the potential field-potential for a ninja student.

The scrolls of Chikamatsu Shigenori contain an Iga tradition that explains how to assess a student's ability to think critically about covert infiltration. The tradition states that the instructor should first show a picture showing a castle to the student and then ask them how they would go about infiltrating it. A student who is not skilled or dull might respond that climbing up the walls would be the best option. The astute student will point out the gate and explain why it is the best way to get in.25 One can imitate others by simply watching how they enter the gate and their dress and mannerisms.

This Yo-nin (see the next section) entry method is not the only option. Instead, the shinobi could use his/her knowledge about locking mechanisms to identify security gaps in door locks and other locks that prevent entry. Although the shinobi could bypass these locks26, it would be considered an In-nin infiltration that could be combined with a Yonin disguise.

Adopting a credulous disguise

Yo-jutsu is the combination of all skills necessary to create a convincing disguise for infiltration. In-jutsu, on the other hand, refers only to those skills that are used in strategic infiltration by exploiting security weaknesses (such sneaking past guards at night).

We can be certain that any mission that required Yo-nin methods had shinobi who carefully selected their clothing for travel to distant or neighboring provinces. They might have been required to blend in with the locals or dress differently depending on the situation. This is why the local dress was preserved and studied.

Shinobi who would be involved in fast-communications as relay runners had to also be able to travel the main-roads. Shinobi were advised to wear reversible clothes so that appearances could be quickly changed.

Black clothing was not recommended for night travel. Moonlit nights require other colors that blend with the environment.

Shinobi dress is closely related to the modern concept of a 'gray man', which means that you don't want to be noticed. Preppers, agents of modern times, and special-forces all use this concept to create a veneer that is easily forgotten by observers. The gray man concept, which is similar to the shinobi art that studies people for the appropriate attire, involves describing the common wear of people in the operating environment.

If a mission requires a specific disguise, it is necessary to create a strong contrast between at most two veneers. Modernizing this principle requires that the clothing be easy to store or trash and in line with cultural behaviors and knowledge. If you don't know the character that you are impersonating, it won't work as disguise. What if the shinobi was questioned about the role he played and didn't know the answers? It would be catastrophic.

To ensure his cover was not exposed, a shinobi learned and imitated the mannerisms, customs and idioms that were appropriate for the disguise he was wearing. This ability is remarkable when you consider that the shinobi not only adopts an outer identity to accomplish a mission but also 'lives the artificial identity.29

A shinobi would need to know the nomenclature for pharmacology in order to be able to mimic a modern doctor or nurse. (What are the side effects and how to administer this medication). He would need to be able to perform all of the clinical skills required by a doctor or nurse. He would also need to be able to identify himself with a fake but reliable form of identification (Hello Dr. 'Pseudonym').

This allowed the shinobi to be flexible in his thinking and actions in order to achieve mission objectives. He was able to recognize that this was an effective deception, and he also learned the right attire and the answers to any questions he might be asked during his mission.

Here is a modern version of the disguise principle. This simply shows how layers of clothing can quickly create a stark contrast between the outer appearance and the inner one.

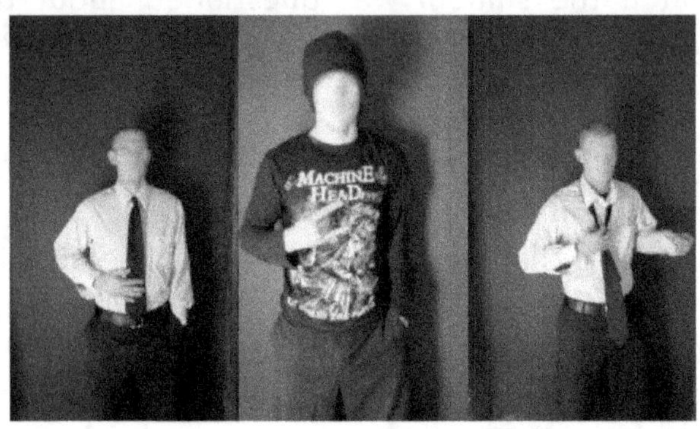

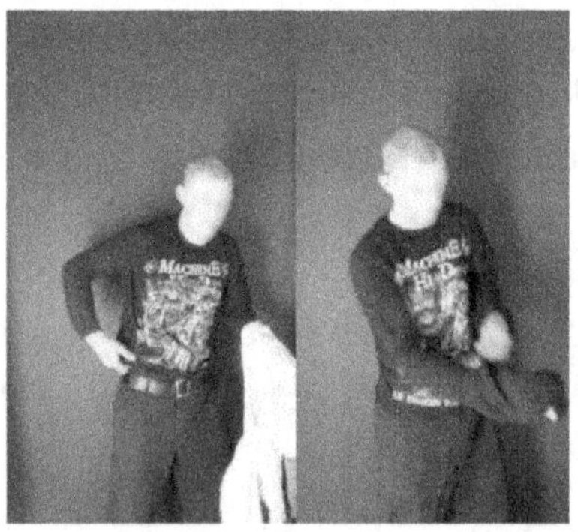

To shift from a "casual business" veneer to a "rock/metal subculture", the business shirt is stripped and the glasses are removed. A carrying bag with props that matches the veneers can be used to create more creative versions.

necessary. This is only a minor version of a flexible.

principle. There is so much more!

There are many factors that go into making a good disguise. These include skills, knowledge and social buoyancy. For a deeper understanding of Yo-nin arts, consult the ninjutsu text.

Ongyo Jutsu: Hide Like a Shinobi

A shinobi has infiltrated an area and succeeded.

He has achieved his goals and now needs a quick fix.

He will not be killed if he retreats. But, oops, the Shinobi

A pursuit ensues after it is spotted. What should you do? What to do?

Shinobi might use a variety tools to throw his shinobi.

Followers can be confused or thrown off the trail.

The popularity of the

bamboo tetsubishi (aka caltrop). These caltrops are a good example of what a caltrop is made of.

Sharp points that, when placed on the escape path, will

Injuring one's feet can deter one's pursuers. According to the Bansenshukai testubishi can be used to deter others from entering a structure.

They fled, but they were out.

The circumstances may dictate that the shinobi might be allowed to practice.

Instead, you can choose to use an alternative escape method by feigning

A plunge into the water. This is simply done by

Cast an arbitrary object in a body water.

Within hearing distance of your enemy.31 This is another way to escape.

It is funny, because you pretend to be one among the alerted

pursuers. This technique must be correctly executed

Shinobi are advised to wear only one color clothing

(brown) Outwardly, and a different colour (grey) Inwardly

During escape, one can change their appearance quickly.

The shinobi should change his clothes while fleeing.

Out and shout to his pursuers that there is a night attack

This can be done while the culprit is giving false directions

escape.32

Controlling the Breath

A habit of controlling one's breathing has been developed.

Itoh described this as the essential first step in ninjutsu

Training.33 This is one reason why training is so important

The regulation of the breath functions in the ability to skillfully.

Art of avoiding detection by enemies and adhering to rules

34 Trainees were told to keep a calm spirit even when faced with adrenaline-educating danger.

Develop the ability to the point that their breath is no longer a problem

35 The method used to do this

The only thing that could be used to cultivate skill is simple breathing

Meditation in which the trainee focuses his attention on a single point below

The navel is used for abdominal breathing with an

Intention to calm the mind. The act of abdominal breathing may become so common that the person no longer needs to think about it. The Shinobi Hiden also mentions another method to reduce the sound of the breath: inserting paper in the mouth and clenching the teeth with it.

Agility and Balance

It is said that to cultivate balance, a felled person must be rehabilitated.

Tree was used by the young trainee as a tool to help him walk and do his chores.

There are many exercises that can be done to maintain equilibrium. You can do these exercises while maintaining equilibrium.

The trainee reached the level of skill that is required to maintain the balance

The beam reached an ever greater height.

This skill probably served a function.

Unusual methods of doing things are a good idea.

Infiltration or espionage. A great balance allows for the ability

to utilize infiltration/espionage routes not recognized by

Those who lack the ability. Balance high up is one example.

A branch from a tree can be used to survey an area.

Natural camouflage provides security.

One should cultivate agility.

Ask yourself why agility is so important.

Agility is about the dexterous movement and coordination of the body.

Human beings are born with a physical body.

It is vital that the body is properly maintained.

The primary way to interact with the

world. Training in physical agility should not be relegated to the backburner.

To the domain of the "fitness club", for within

These establishments are merely machines, but they can also be used to exercise.

Equipment to improve the strength of the muscles

and joints. The "movements" of the machines are taught to the user

and instructors of fitness, rather than creative movements

Expressions that are offensive or defensive in nature. One could go to the gym and do squats.

You can do leg presses up to the point that your legs are raw muscle. However, this person won't be able to run up a wall regardless of his/her physical condition. This skill requires physical agility, which can only be achieved through consistent practice and a clear goal. It is important that you understand the differences between agility and physical fitness.

Jumping from High Places

Hicho no Tsutae, a Koka Ninja tradition, is described

Shigenori to reduce injury risk

The impact of a fall from high places or jump from them.

Shinobi are instructed to use a sword or staff.

When you jump from a height, scabbard should be in such a manner that it is not visible.

The scabbard and staff should first impact the ground

By doing so, you absorb and distribute the weight of the

38 The physics of properly receiving the ground

A height is all about force distribution. If one does not

Use any implement according to the classic method

It is possible to still practice receiving the ground without any hands.

Jumping from high places requires you to land feet

First, collapse your upper and lower bodies into yourself.

So that you absorb the impact (preferably rolling).

Instead of putting the energy of the falls into one part, deposit it in another.

The body that could cause injury should be treated.

Receive as much information as you can from as many parts of your body.

The ground.

You can start by jumping from a small area.

Height (3') and cement to muscle memory the mechanics

Receiving the ground. This can be used over time.

Ability to leap from great heights, such as one story.

more.

Strengthening your upper-body strength

A warrior may have great physical strength. It is possible to say that physical fitness can be one of the most important factors in predicting the outcome.

A shinobi way trainee would likely engage in many "unconventional" exercises to increase strength and endurance of the upper body. Manual suspension in high places is one example of such unusual exercises. To develop the arms and hands, a trainee could be suspended from a tree for up to an hour.

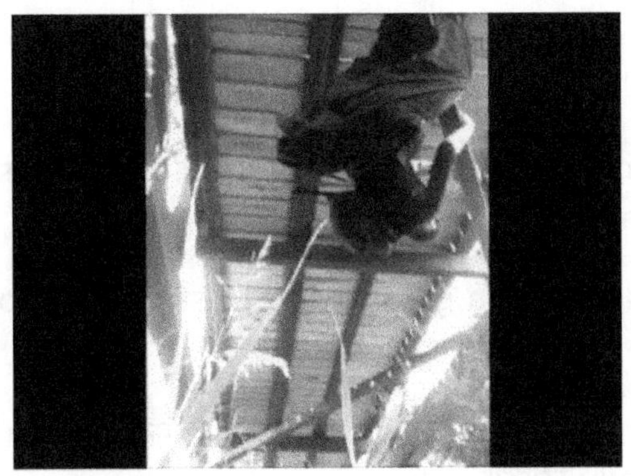

If you are looking for a similar method to build strength, there are many modern options available, such as climbing trees or suspending yourself from under a bridge.

Dislocation of the Joints

40

Swimming

You will also need to learn how to navigate the terrain

The trainee became very proficient in the task quietly.

Swimming silently is an activity. Further observations have been made about it.

Draeger said that the Ninja could swim with enough ease.

His/her legs were so strong that it wasn't at all difficult to write while

Swimming.41 You can easily replicate this skill by using an

A local pool is a great place to start your journey as an enthusiast.

A body of water in which one can swim using their own technique

To practice this, you can use your legs only while keeping your hands up.

satisfaction.

Manufacture, Deployment and Maintenance of Explosives & Incendiaries

The manuals show that shinobi had a good knowledge of how to use explosives and incendiary gadgets.

These devices are primitive and usually call for potassium nitrate. However, they should still be considered as deadly weapons if used correctly.

The majority of explosive device types are hand-grenades or landmines. These devices typically function with a basic black mixture of potassium, sulfur and ash. Incendiaries, on the other hand, include quick-lit torch of various shapes and sizes, as well as airborne missiles (such flaming Arrows) and quick-lit torches.

The Bansenshukai notes that the hand-grenade could be used to inflict diversionary stimulation on the enemy by detonating it during night raids. The proper detonation could help the allies to achieve a successful escape or victory, or be used for other purposes.

The final structure resembles a sphere. It consists of two clay hemispheres, each with large hollowed centers. These hollows are then circumscribed by eight smaller hollows filled with charcoal. The hollow in the center is filled with shot, ignition powder, and iron fillings. The center hollow is filled with ignition powder, shot, and iron fillings.

Self-Immolation

If an Iga shinobi from the past ever felt it necessary,

Kill him/herself. It is recommended that a futon should be prepared by

It should be circumscribed with black powder. The shinobi would set

The room is filled with fires and the futon is used as a suicide bed. The

The black powder would be ignited by the ensuing fires.

44

Surveillance and Espionage

Referring to the espionage skillsets of ninjutsu

Families may have a deeper understanding of what it means

To be a ninja, you can use the term "kancho" This word appears in

The question and answer section in the Bansenshukai

Its significance for the people of Ninjutsu. If you ask about the origin of the

Fujibayashi provides a definition of term and its usage.

The term is broken into two characters: Kan = gap

Or opening; Cho = detect.45 This may lead one to conclude that a shinobi is specialized in exploiting weaknesses in enemy defenses. An immaculate ability to observe is a prerequisite for assessing an enemy's defenses.

Indeed, the shinobi were very skilled in this area. Shochu Kokorozuke no Koto, for example, is an example of this art.

Transmitted in the writings by Chikamatsu Shigenori

Gunpo Jiyoshu46 that explains the phenomenon is alluded to

It is important to observe the insects around you.

Shigenori tells a story about two to illustrate the art.

Shinobi who were made aware of one another's presence by The

Activities of the insects in the vicinity. The story continues

One shinobi tried to penetrate the building.

An ally shinobi was awoken by the sudden onset of

He was notified by mosquito movement that he should

Stop infiltration The shinobi who occupy the

Quarters heard the gradual decline in cricket sounds.

He was alerted to the possibility of an infiltrating Shinobi.

Truth Assessment

One could sum up a human comparison.

It is comparable to any other species known, so it is reasonable

To conclude that the most important aspects of the human being are

Being's evolution in terms of adaptation

The human mind is the source of defensiveness and offensiveness.

To make a person innocuous in all respects.

One must simply devise a way to deprive a person

Being able to think or utterly confuse its mind

As to the nature and reality of truth. To

If one satisfies this purpose, it makes good sense to use.

deception.

This is why a shinobi should have been armed

With the tools necessary to assess the truth of certain

Information that could be collected during the course of

intelligence operations. These tools: What could they be?

Answer: The principles and logic of reason.

Truth can only be achieved by applying the right principles.

Principles of Reason. These are the first two: logic and reasoning. Logic is the first.

Science concerned with the flow or soundness of

Conclusions from supporting premises Logic,

"Learns us laws and principles through which we can."

You can test the accuracy of any piece or reasoning using our

"Other person's or your own." 48The science of logic is today

Complex validation requires many rules to follow

Refutation or confirmation of truth. To the shinobis of old, however, these are rudiments

Logic was likely to be crucial in the identification

propaganda.

The 4th volume in the Shinobi Hiden is an example.

The reader is instructed to be cautious about any information they receive

Directly or indirectly, from an enemy source To

It is possible to establish a value for truth regarding such information.

It is recommended that the shinobi engages in a logical dissection

The material is characterized by a search to find contradictions or

Inconsistencies that are expressed by other people

49

Situations that require a shinobi to assess truth

It was no surprise that the task required a lot of observation skills.

A single detail missing could be detrimental to your project.

Final conclusion.

The Network

Uncontrolled information about yourself is the most dangerous for personal security. The collection and analysis of information about something is what gives rise to actionable intelligence.

In order to keep an eye on the enemy's activities, huge information networks were created by sending shinobi to various locations.50 They engaged in activities that brought them in contact with many people to expand the network's reach over time.

These shinobi arrived at the designated area in accordance to a tradition that recommends that they map the area mentally by walking and watching.51 This helped them build a wealth of knowledge that would help him achieve his goals.

The Bansenshukai have shown that the secret information networks of shinobi could have been expanded to include other types of agents with varying purposes, including female agents52 (kunoichi), children53, and local residents.

How to steer the enemy

One ninjutsu principle is known as

Suigetsu No Daiji (The Principle of the Moon and Water)

An enemy spy who successfully penetrated allied forces

Not to be killed and rooted out, but instead to be considered

As a potential asset.

Converting the enemy is all that is required

Spy to support the cause of the allies. It's easy enough. To do

This is why one should show generosity

Kindness to enemy spy, including provision of clothes

Money, food, and advice about what is best for him

interest. This principle can be used to spy on the enemy.

You may eventually develop sympathies that lead to conversion.

Depending on the situation, this may allow for the provision of the

Allies forces are a valuable tool.

Ura-awase No Daiji (Principle Of) is another principle.

Secret Connection) detailed by Chikamatsu in his writings

Shigenori makes allusions to cognitive acumen

The Shinobi on the propagation and dissemination of disinformation

Use of psychological techniques to enlist enemy forces

probabilities.

When applied correctly, the principle consists of

Purposively inciting anger and dissatisfaction among an

Allies spy. He should be angry at the side he serves

thereby be less loyal to its cause. The allied forces eventually won.

Spy must hear a plan to defeat enemy forces

Although it sounds plausible, the actual story is a hoax. His grudge.

The allied spy may desire to 'get' against his master, lord, etc.

"Back" at the person who has angered you, to be precise. This is the idea.

Get the begrudged spy on your side to reveal information about a "secret program"

To the enemy side.

If the operation is successful, the enemy might not be

So quick to act upon the information provided by the Allies Spy.

Shadowy source (how can you trust a Ninja? As such, the

The Koka tradition, according to the principle, is the propagation

You can make disinformation more convincing by making a prisoner your prisoner.

Perhaps from the enemy's side to hear about some "secret"

plan". The prisoner will then be able to access the conduit.

Make his escape should be provided in a way that seems to make sense

accidental. The prisoner may then seek out the enemy.

The "secret plan" will be revealed.

The enemy forces could then act in accordance.

With the disinformation provided, the allied can be allowed to

Forces can win a decisive victory if they know in advance

It is precisely what the enemy will do.55

The Iga tradition of this principle is imitated by the

Same with one variable being altered - plan should

It should be real, and it should seem that the allied forces actually are

It is difficult to keep it secret.

It is believed that the secret was spread after rumors were circulated.

The enemy intelligence network will pick it up

Chatter and plan accordingly. This is the "secret" plan.

You must be aware that you may lose an ally.

You may have to incur some expenses, but it is not for nothing.

Once this trick has been tried a few more times, it's finally over.

The enemy will soon become used to hearing rumors

Real plans. This gives the enemy the confidence to take advantage of the allies.

side.

Another rumor about a "secret" will surface when the time is right.

Plan" should be propagated only if the plan is in its final form.

Fake it. When the enemy acts in confidence,

Their intelligence gathered false information

Networks, the allied forces will have an advantage

You can anticipate the actions of your enemy and be able to react accordingly

56

Good Cop

Protect an area from the actions of enemies

Shinobi: It was recommended that one openly hire someone well-known to be a shinobi

Shinobi, and make it public. This was done.

It is a deterrent to enemy activities

Sending the message that the province has been monitored One can also increase security by

Hidden shinobi are used to monitor the activities

Province.57 These agents should be referred to

Yo no Shinobi (not hidden), and In no Shinobi [hidden].

Fidelity Assessment

A mission was undertaken to retrieve the items.

Information is important, so one should be wary of his/her own spy.

What if they have converted and are now attempting to deceive?

You with false information? This Chikamatsu can be prevented

Writes of Kaeri toi no Koto: The art of asking questions

spies.

Traditions of art are the reason for the warning that

One should not ask a shinobi for the information.

Collect from a mission with other shinobi.

This is done to stop the group of shinobi being expelled.

Hearing is the best way to keep a lie straight through hearing

Each other. Instead, it is better to question each shinobi individually. Then compare the information to determine if there are any contradictions.

suspicion concerning a shinobi's loyalty.

Traditions also indicate that you can make up stories

Then, ask the shinobi questions about what it is.

To drive out indicators of the, it is completely false

Existence of disloyalty.58

Relay Runners

In the event that shinobi were located far from each other,

How did they transmit messages secretly to one another?

From one area to another?

Answer: There's an Iga Ninja tradition.

A team of ordinary people could be used as messengers.

To facilitate the quick, they are geographically separated at specific intervals.

Transmission of information in one area to another

"urgent" situations. This is the translation

Tradition derives provides few details about all

What specific methods and tools are needed for this?

One could however imagine many successes in a successful operation

Potential nuances are allowed provided the principle underpinning the

Tradition simply refers to the ability to send messages using a different method than usual.

The enemy is aware.

Before we can explain the principle behind this

The modern world can benefit from the wisdom of tradition,

A basic understanding of the historical must be acquired

context that is related to this tradition.

During the Sengoku Jidai era of medieval Japan

As power became more fragmented, geographic regions were fractured.

Shifted from clans to tribes, and family to family. With so many

Influential powers vie for the seat at universal control

It was important that you listened to all the happenings of

For better preparation, be sure to visit neighboring provincials

A decision concerning troop movements, or dissolving

alliances. Cummins and Koka Ninja Skills are related to the fact that Kimura Yasutaka's younger brother, the ninja master at Koka who had previously taught Shigenori Koka techniques, once served in the capacity of messenger for Owari-Tokugawa clan. Kimura Kogoemon was his given name. In his Owari Tokugawa clan service he reported to him on a potential rebellion at Mt. Koya Region in 1692. The intelligence report, which was said to have been provided by a Koka network, was to inform his master on whether to send troops in the region or determine whether the rebellion would be strengthened by more Ronin. This communicated the existence of a serious problem.

Regional stability

Before the advent satellites, fiber-optic cables, and satellites

Systems and information concerning distant lands were

acquired by the five senses and abilities of a spy; an shinobi. Once

Obtained, the data would not normally be

The speed of light is not used, though smoke and firesignals are sometimes used. It's the speed of a horse.

human being, but sometimes at the speed and agility of an arrow. The ninjutsu tradition utilizing 'tsugihikyaku' (or

The relay runners then staff information networks.

The common use of peasants (peasant workers) was included in the constitution.

Not only can you transmit messages from allied provinces but also from them.

territories. The relay would consist primarily of messengers

who were separated at irregular intervals and would operate beneath

They were claiming to be communicating market prices.

Provincial goods. If they were not allowed to continue,

Their intentions were well concealed and they were not being truthful when they were questioned.

message was preserved.59

In today's information-rich world, there is no shortage of information

The internet makes it easy to send messages across the globe using technology

You can travel the entire planet in one blink. It is important to note that this does not include the fact that

Capability is convenient. It carries with itself a certain amount

security risk. One should assume that any

Electronic transmission of any kind of information is possible

You can log information somewhere, or you can find a way to break the security of these digital mediums. To transmit information over long distances, without suspicion or leaving a digital record, and to maintain highest levels of information security, one can use pre-modern intelligence methods like

Relay runners.

It's the same with any message spoken verbally.

A message between parties can be subject to communication

to the fragilities human subjectivity. You can always play the

Do you like to play telephone games? If so, at one time you have

Have you experienced the loss of communication?

it bears a close resemblance the original. This understanding will allow you to

It is evident that the messengers have to be loyal.

The information they receive must be verified.

How fast could this system be implemented in such low tech?

What message was expected to travel among runners? Given the

Itoh's research proved that messengers could travel 60 to 70 miles.

There are miles to go in a day. But for shorter distances, it is more time.

Depending on the speed of a runner, it could be even faster.

Infiltration and diversion

To infiltrate a country, one could even

Iga means a compound or fortress used to spy.

Koka traditions from Yamabiko (echoes), suggest that the

It is best to approach the target with a diversion strategy.

If you're not taking full advantage of the flank, it is better to start from one point.

The enemy forces

This tradition is found in Chikamatsu's text

derived does not provide information on diversion

should be used or for what purpose. But, where to put it?

The tradition in the text is next to the principles for Shinobi

to be used in infiltrating another province, it indicates

Yamabiko may also have been used infiltration.

It would be one example of a diversion.

Any other method should be used, but one shouldn't approach from the

The diversion point should be approached in an opposite direction. 60

A Linguist

If the operation required that one venture to another province

In these cases, the local residents spoke in a different dialect

There are other problems than those to which the shinobi was trained.

The possibility of problems in the execution or implementation of a plan may arise. The locals might be willing to help.

Please note the local tongue used by the shinobi

Thus, we can make an assessment of whether he is an agent or worse.

That would be too difficult for the shinobi.

was communicated to parties of interested who are

Conversations were had. It was therefore deemed

It is important that shinobi have a command of the local environment.

The skill of speaking dialects is comparable to modern-day skills

Intelligence agents who are required to travel internationally as part of their job

duties.

Haruhiko kindaichi, linguist.

The book The Japanese Language describes regional differences.

Dialects were and are still "conspicuous", lending a reason to

Believe the shinobi had plenty of work to do in achieving their goal.

fluency:

"The everyday conversations that people have with each other"

Kagoshima's prefecture cannot even be understood by Kumamoto's neighbor, nor those on Honshu or Shikoku.

Kindaichi comments that to illustrate the difficulty of linguistic matters for the shinobi, it is not uncommon for a regional dialect be encrypted or confused in order to stop infiltration by ninja.

"[D]uring the feudal years, the Satsuma Clan deliberately made the speech its domain unintelligible and visible to outsiders in order for them to be safe from the Shogunate's spies."62

It was considered a talent that a shinobi had mastered the regional dialects and traveled extensively throughout the world and within his country.

This is yet again a reflection of what is expected in candidates who want to become modern Intelligence operatives.

UdeKarami, Enervating The Enemy

In ninjutsu books, it is evident that the shinobi took matters of travel within and between the provinces seriously. They used appropriate cover to hide their identities. This allowed them to appear on well-trodden roads like merchants, common travelers, and monks. Their trade involved mortal danger if they were known to send communications against the lord. This aspect of Ninjutsu was so important that it was prized enough by opposing Lords to make use of their own Shinobi to stop spies from entering their lands.

They might have been in a dangerous situation, where the enemy could pursue them if they had lost their artificial veneer. So what would we expect of a ninja who was being pursued by an enemy soldier or foot-soldier and was forced to tether him?

You can't limit the resourcefulness of ninjutsu to just a few options. He could throw out thorny, sharp caltrops that could be used to attack the feet and others following him; he can race off into the darkness to escape their shadowy depths or fix fuses in trees to confuse his trail; but the one technique we will cover today would most likely have been done during the daylight hours to protect a single enemy whose goal was to track the spy who had been identified.

Ude Karami 64is defined by the use of one's swordscabbard as psychological deterrent against followingers. It is quite simple to use or as easy as we can get from the texts. The tail saw the scabbard and was immediately alerted by it being on the ground. The escape-seeking shinobi was still making his escape.

You can think about it. It is possible to imagine a time when everyone was happy.

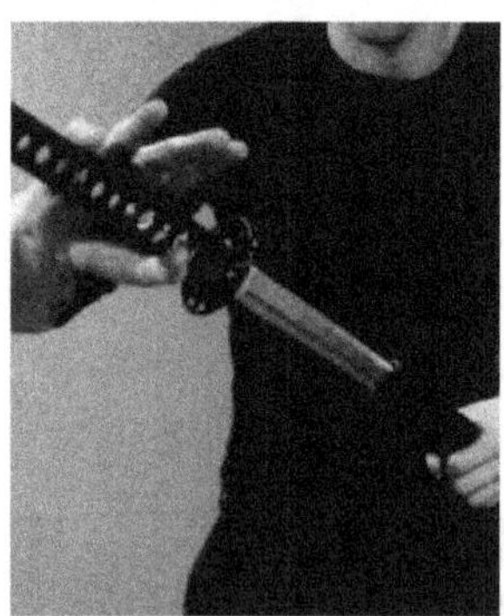

Armaments could include swords or bows and and arrows as well as spears or pikes. Anybody who saw a scabbard laid on the ground such as this must have been cautious. This tactic could have been quite successful in giving the evading shinki more time to create distance between them.

Chapter 6: The Occult Pragms And Philosophy Of

The Ninja

Itoh describes Iga's and Koka's ninja as being bushi warriors/samurai. Their skills were developed through years of battle between the various clans. In the beginning, Iga, Koka, and other clans were adversaries. This fact is supported by their history as frequent rivalries.

The Iga's and Koka's predecessors to the Ninja were known to have used methods of mountain navigation and region surveillance during this period to engage in war with neighbouring families. It is because of this period of infighting that it is possible to question the morality and integrity of the ninja.

Sengoku Era saw the men from Iga, Koka and their reputations in spying which led to important military victories.

Ninja could not associate themselves with acts that did no reflect the integrity or strength of a warrior after the Sengoku Era became the Edo Era. It was necessary to preserve their noble, earned status. Therefore, any ninja who was associated with a theftster had to be extinguished.

Morality, the Bansenshukai

It is evident that the contents include

There are many options available to help you achieve your goals.

Fujibayashi, empowerment of the common criminal

Recognized need for a guiding spirit

3. Titled Philosophy within the First Chapter of His Manual.

'Seishin' (correct mind), the chapter cautions the reader

The practitioner of Ninjutsu must keep the appropriate

You can see their mindset in all they do. This is the essence of correctness in mind

It is defined as a belief in what is "righteous", loyal, or good.

"Benevolent" can also mean offering an opportunity for the

Presupposes the one is "gentle and kind."

Respecting these virtues is the only contradiction.

This literature must be mentioned because it concerns the

The loyalty of a Shinobi to a Lord

Zoughari claimed that Zoughari made this statement during the Kamakura

Period (1192-1333 AD).

Ideals of loyalty that they were more concerned in

There is no other way to pay for their services than through battle recognition.4

This idea is clearly contrary to what has already been written

Fujibayashi. In the Bansenshukai, he states in several

Shinobi must practice a strong level of discretion in certain places

Loyalty one's lord.5,6,7 Stephen K. Hayes does not agree with the

Fujibayashi & Zoughari's claims regarding declaring that

Shinobi were more focused on the preservation of their ancestral land.

Families rather than their relationships with feudal Lords.8

What is the truth about this?

The Bansenshukai: A compendium of many Iga

Koka traditions, certainly should be considered a reliable

Consider the fact that the source was written by the author.

The history is closer than you think, but in the words one man has to say

It is important not to forget one aspect of history.

contradictions.

Hayes' claim to familial loyalty was cited.

It is also important to mention that the manual Fujibayashi has many other aspects.

This admonishes you to maintain a image of non-affiliation

As the times required, you can also use any of these shinobi arts.

A family member might be able serve the interests

Contrary to the shinobi, a lord. The historical

Zoughari records show that not every ninja is equal

Their lord was their greatest loyalty, but they would not turn on them.

Allegiances are made if there is a compelling reason to do so. Although it is possible to be a virtue,

Loyalty in the manual was only pontificated

In order to make ninjutsu more honorable.

Whatever the truth, there's no contradiction

exists.

Respect for the virtues that are found in the

Bansenshukai may be asked where they came from

Which translations have they been observed into human?

conduct?

The Five include two of these virtuous principled.

Virtues and practices of Esoteric Buddhism that are also known under the name "the"

Confucianism has five precepts. These virtues have been described

Kukai is a monk

"The virtues of kindness, righteousness and propriety are the five virtues. The term 'not-killing' is used to describe 'benevolence'. It refers to treating others the way you would want them to be treated.

'Righteousness means 'not taking,' which means that you must save and give to others. Propriety is an acronym for 'not committing infidelity'. It also means to observe all five rites. Wisdom is defined as 'not taking intoxicants'. This means that you make wise decisions and think well. Sincerity can be a synonym to 'not lying.' It is the ability to act on one's words without hesitation.

The Ego, and a Higher Cause

Shinobi eventually found motivation in their endeavors.

A value system which distinguished them from other endeavors

to criminals and rogue Assassins and kept them in

They are often samurai and fellow shinobi. In fact,

It is possible for an individual to call themselves a shinobi

When you have the skills of ninjutsu at your disposal,

This is contrary to what is.

Written in Bansenshukai

Fujibayashi Yasutake - the man who wrote down the 17th

century shinobi book makes warnings that anyone can do it.

Individual who tries ninjutsu as a means to get rich

The end result will be disastrous.10

Itoh observes that admonition matches Itoh's observation.

In the defense of the state, ninjutsu was employed. Accordingly to the ninja tradition, the strictest moral code was required. To anyone who attempted to profit by using ninjutsu it was said that this would eventually lead to harm.

to the user.11

This is because the universal causality explains it all.

Everything that is now known about the universe, has its origins in

In accordance with the motivational laws that underlie these principles

"Righteousness"," "fidelity", "benevolence", "loyalty", and other related terms.

Fujibayashi says that these principles are essential.

be observed and respected so that they are inextricably

Associated with the Ways Of Heaven, and so to

They are to be contradicted.

It god, gods "Buddha", and any other deified ascriptions of the

One can pray to universal causality.12Fujibayashi

With polemical prose it is hard to ignore these

Principles to support sensory stimulation for humanity

You are most likely to want to act in accordance to the way the

shinobi. It is the best way to ensure you are on the right path.

It is imperative that the tempting temptations to the senses are not allowed to influence you.

reciprocated. One must also not attempt to indulge.

oneself.13

These facts support the idea of ninjutsu

It was once the art for the self-less that could only be achieved through the

Eliminating the self-interest that is at root of ego

What is the best way for a shinobi to keep his discipline in the gym?

Face to face with execution, torture, and all facets of mission which

In tandem, mental and physically tough required great mental resilience

A loyalty unwavering to one's Lord.

This is why it can be argued the elimination of

Positive social implications of one's own ego can speak volumes about your ability to communicate with others.

The purpose and role of the shinobi in peace and war. The death

Ego is the birth into a domain or state of being.

The self-interests are ignored. This is the way to be.

Supports the society's collective burdens with a strength

This is what a selfish individual would never be able to possess. Because the Shinobi's purpose was to protect the society through any means necessary, including self sacrifice, it should not be forgotten that he suffered vicariously. He gave his entire life to the welfare and well-being of others. This lifestyle could not possibly be understood to reflect the highest ideals of living.

You are a criminal.

Although there are likely to be shinobi out there who did,

Incongruent, immoral, and egregious acts

With some ninjutsu traditional principles.

These types of Shinobi should not, however, be considered.

Master representatives are the embodiment of what ninjutsu means. Zoughari is the controversial Togakure Ryu.

That the essence of Ninjutsu cannot be taught is an important fact

Only the few individuals who have the "deepest humanity"

"Quality"15, but despite this allusion it is still compassionate

You should know the benevolent masters ninjutsu.

To inflict injury, the authentic traditions of the shinobi were directed

Whoever challenges their authority is doomed to death.

prerogatives.

Fujibayashi says, for example that the killings are a matter of principle.

The saving of many people from an indecent person is justified.

This is in accordance with "benevolence".16

Principle, he says is the act of showing compassion to all

This principle should be followed.

Take down the person who robs the welfare

many.17

This concern for "good" in the collective might be

What drove the shinobi's determination to destroy anyone who opposed him?

Could have compromised a mission, innocuous or not. After

All, the shinobi of ancient times were engaged in a militant

A polarized atmosphere can lead to a loss of sense of right or wrong.

It was their duty to protect their lords, and his people. The

This was done to count the weight of a single life as insignificant

Comparatively to the thousands of lives he has impacted

Protective.

This is what it says in the translated works

Chikamatsu Chigenori on the subject Iga und Koka Ninja

Traditions hold that it's acceptable and necessary that a shinigi be present

Every person who learns a secret not to be kept must be killed

divulged.18

In-Yo & the Five Elements

The world was known to the ancient shinobi

Through an applied understanding of duality - a notion that is

You can find it across cultures. It's white and it's black, up and downstairs.

These qualitative descriptions can be empty or filled.

Many phenomena have been witnessed by the shinobi

The result was a classification of opposites.

functioned through the definitions "In" and "Yo".19

The origins of Japanese In-Yo are unknown.

While it is difficult to pinpoint the exact cause, one could say that the phenomenon is "a common phenomenon".

Nuance of Chinese concept of "yin-yang".

Alongside the in-yo classification of world items

Fujibayashi refers in this instance to the Go-Dai

Origins of the alchemical theory can be traced back to antiquity.

Tsou believed to have first described it

Yen (350 to 270 BC).20 This theory comes from Buddhism

explains the universal processes that are the result

The interaction between five different energies is called:

Wood, Fire, Earth, Metal, Water.

Hayes doesn't describe the Go-Dai he refers to, however.

Earth, Water, Fire, Air/wind, Void/ space

Hayes refers here to the Go Dai of Japanese Esoteric Buddhism. It includes an additional sixth animating aspect - the mind.

Death and Life

Fujibayashi asserts that the "primary principles" from which all of form, including existence, comes is emptiness. Because one's being is composed of various combinations of the Five Elements (earth and water, fire, metal and wood), the shinobi should understand that his essence cannot be separated from the womb. With this understanding, the shinobi can let go of attachment to the earth and fear of dying. His death and life are one and same in relation the primary principle. This understanding allows the shinobi to let go of any fear or attachment to the material world and to accept death with open arms.

Fujibayashi elaborates further on the truths about death and living, explaining with poetic prose that 'death' is actually an abstract illusion. For all things, whether they are manifest or not, nothing truly dies. All of them, however, are interconnected. They all arise from and dissolve back in the substance that is blood of the universe. This is why the form of everything will not end but instead will endure the trials and tribulations of the universe until the end. They are only divided because of the mind's obsessions with duality. This insight enabled the shinobi not only to forget his attachment to death and fear, but also to transcend the limitations of existential inquests. He could live in accordance the will the universe.

Fujibayashi's book on ninjutsu, "Determinism and The Determination of Die," is a recurring theme

This is an example of a deterministic philosophical belief. It was his belief, or perhaps it was the belief of other Shinobi, that every individual at conception is forever bound to a destiny that oozes from universal law.24 One should not forget that regardless of one's choices in life, they will all end in the same way. This is the way that the laws of nature are. Any attempt at escaping these laws is to seek to become free of them.

existence.

Let's take as an example the method by which a tree is propagated.

The tree bears fruits and grows. The potential for all that is possible with a

One plant is already determined from the seeds.

It grows. One can help increase the growth rate

Good soil and adequate sunlight are essential, but you must also ensure that there is no mucking around.

No matter how many choices there are in taking care of your dog, it doesn't matter.

No one can stop the inevitable of death.

The plant will grow and mature throughout its life.

The environment can have an impact on the fruit's quality, but it doesn't matter how they are grown.

We might have to force it (except if we don't want the thing to live to start).

You can't do without it, because your potential is already known. Human life is like that. There are many things we can do.

You can take this or that route, but you're ludicrous.

Believing that we have control of our lives. Sometimes, we may even be able to.

Medical technology can help us alter our genetic predispositions.

Gene therapy, which allows you to extend your life span with gene therapy, is one example of such a technique.

number of years you can enjoy. But regardless of our choices,

we make, we might never escape death. It is always there

lurking.

Accepting the possibility of death is the best way to go.

Now!

Shugendo

What spiritual practices might have assisted the healing?

Shinobi, the elimination of the mind or the development

Fujibayashi's Seishin? A Seishin for Fujibayashi?

Shugendo is a way to 'train and develop your mind' in relative isolation.

Testing 26 is a religion founded by the mountain monk, En

No Gyoja (634-706 A.D.), has been characterized in this way:

Blend between Shintoism/Buddhism.27,28

Man, many Ninjutsu practitioners, some once peasant

Farmers became immersed in the difficult work of agriculture.

Shugendo should absorb the knowledge of the Yama-bushi

(mountain Ascetics - A person who trains in mountains

This was thought to be an incredible source of supernatural energy

power.29 It is true to its name, the religion enjoys a good reputation.

Its harsh "shugyo", an oriented method of spiritual refinement

One could describe it as a constant test on one's inner.

and outside strength.

Indeed, Shugendo monks practice(d) many rituals

The test would determine one's limit to death, and display to.

The observer experiences a certain degree physical difficulty.

Only the devoted can survive. One example:

Practice includes a winter seclusion away from technology

Comforts high above the mountains. This is what it's done with

The ultimate goal of obtaining special spiritual powers.

The ability to walk through heat and expose oneself.

insult of boiling waters.30

to be proofs of the reality of attained supernatural

Powers, however, to be certain, the implications of such an

This observation could be subject to discussion. This debate may be discussed.

It was in reference to the ninjas practitioners of the Kuji.

Kevin Keitoshi Casey made this observation in his book The Ninja Mind.

The particulars weren't of interest to the ninja.

There were no details on how the rituals worked for the kuji, but they were

Thought to approach the matter kuji using a sense

Pragmatism, which focuses on ascertaining reality

The question of whether rituals could help in the development

Great power.31

Shugyos and Shugendos for the Ninja

Shugendo pilgrimages involve physical labor

The pilgrimages are not for everyone.

Achieve success by understanding their physical limitations

but also a mental attitude to allow for advancement

Human potential – A key attribute to the

Composition of the historical ninja.

This is probably the most challenging part of Shugendo instruction.

Okugake, a type of pilgrimage. This pilgrimage consists of

A foot-based route covering 80 kilometers.

It takes just a few days to get from one mountain to another. The route is

People tend to find it treacherous and difficult to forgive.

Every year, there is something missing from the pilgrimage trail.32

Shugendo why should one subject the

Are you unable to bear such an extreme difficulty? Answer: These Shugenja (one who

Shugendo, or practices Shugendo), were heroes of their respective societies

Communities who suffered for the greater benefit of others

Their fellow human beings. Their ventures and hermitage

Nature has always been there with the intent to endure.

Get knowledge and power in the spirit realm.

could be used to protect the community.33

Although this may sound obvious, it is not something that was widely known.

These are some of the ways to tell if you have a mental illness.

Attitude, which has been affixed the public perception

Shinobi.

This connection of Shugendo and Ninjutsu could be

Further supported by the writings Of Itoh

Ninjutsu was described by some as a way to deepen spiritual and emotional connection.

Practitioners are left with a sense of physical conditioning.

The determination to endure even the most difficult situations

"Brutal" of life-events.34

Intensifying your mental and spiritual well-being was the goal

Shagyo or "tanren" is a method to condition the mind.

Exposure to harsh elements and extreme physical challenges can expose the body to "challening" conditions.

training.

Another link between Shugendo (ninjutsu)

What is known as "the kuji shin ho" of practices

ninjutsu. This kuji ho is an occult technique of selfprotection. It involves various hand positions.

Concentrated intentions and intertwinements

(mandalas), spoken vows and mantras (mantras), are believed to have spiritual meanings.

Increase one's ability to be sensitive to the surrounding environment

35It is important to note that within the

Shugendo rituals have a method of

Demon exorcism commonly known as "the kuji Jiu Zi" ceremony

Nine mudras and 9 formulas are used to draw the attention of the

Power of supernatural gods"36. This fact demonstrates an

Influence of ritual on the Kuji Goshin Ho

Shugendo also includes a ritual.

This is commonly known as 'Takigyo' and is used to purify your mind.

By standing under the torrent of a, you can get rid of all negativity.

Chanting mantras while chanting and freezing waterfall are some of the ideas.

To invoke the powers 'kami.

Koshikidake asserts that the "kuji in", which consists of

Of performing nine specific intertwinements in the hands

Along with invoking a specific mental state, you can also use your fingers.

The idea is that it can be used before you enter the waterfall.37

The association of the kuji toshin ho and ninjutsu is called the

Mountain religion should be treated as a speculative belief.

However, it is not a mere notion. It can also be used for other purposes.

Modern ninjutsu practitioners should be noted

Practices that reflect their heritage are still being followed

Shugendo roots. Koshikidake is one example.

Casey's texts regarding Shugendo and kuji,

Stephen K. Hayes, in full Shugenja attire

What appears to be an 'Taikgyo' ritual.

Kuji In & Ninjutsu

The author might not be able to provide any information about the origins or the history of the kuji kushin ho. It is fascinating to note, however, that the nine fingers entwined in the ninjutsu goshinh have a very exact resemblance of the Nine Esoteric Seals of Buddhist Qui-gong38. The origin of these nine spoken command characters was set in 4th century writings of master Ge Hong39.

This Buddhist influence validates that the teachings about the Kuji originated in China over a thousand centuries ago. Francois Lepine a Kuji-In practitioner, states in his book Advanced Kuji-In the claim that the Kuji rituals originate with Hinduism (India) and are later transported to China.

The Romanized vows of both the Japanese and Chinese command characters are compared here.

Nine Jumon Voweds of Ninjutsu's Kuji Goshin ho = Rin. Pyo. Toh. Sha. Kai. Jin. Retsu. Zai.

Nine Command Characters from the Baopuzi by Gehong = Lin Bing Dou Zhe Jie Zhen Lie Zai Qian.

Baopuzi's nine command character characters serve the same purpose as the ninja's Jumon vows. Lepine, on contrary, claims that the purpose for practicing the kuji was to attain self-knowledge.

Although kuji can be used by others, Hatsumi acknowledges that it is possible to use it for other purposes. Hatsumi says that the primary functions of the "ninja"'s kuji rituals can be carried out by those who have not had experience or training in the occult.

Kuji practice

Stephen K. Hayes. Francois Lapine. Kevin

Keitoshi casey believes the kuji should not be

This information cannot be gleaned from text alone, it can only by learned

under the direction of a competent teacher.45.46

If this is true, someone who has read the literature might have done so.

The following questions were raised.

First, who was first to teach the original preceptor?

ninja's kuji ritual? Deep knowledge is, therefore, essential

Development takes time and, in some instances, generations.

This clarified knowledge should be passed on to competent teachers

This may be necessary when instructing a student at the kuji.

However, this should not be taken to mean that one is able to assume.

A competent teacher is essential to learn the kuji.

Acquisition of deep knowledge concerning the kuji

The accuracy of the results has not been confirmed without the guidance and support of a teacher. Hatsumi of Togakure has seconded his statement

In 1988, he stated that he would not reveal the secrets to anyone.

The ninja's "kuji" until his/her taijutsu became perfect.

He believes that excellence is what is needed.

The kuji had been preceptorship before he was able to do so.

That would be better than pretending that the kuji doesn't exist.

You don't need to be a candidate, because you won't get the one you want.

47. Hatsumi further explains that

The essence kuji doesn't just belong to ninjutsu.

Training and showing how physically inexplicable it is

There are actions that can connote supernatural power such as moving

Out of the way for an incoming punch that one doesn't understand,

People can perform this task without any prior training.

Awareness of the role of the Kuji.48 Hatsumi adds that nobody has the ability to teach the kuji teachings. Hatsumi, however, states that Stephen K. Hayes did not receive his kuji instruction from Hatsumi. This author will not pursue trivialities but encourages you to look for the answer if it interests you.

We now turn our attention to the content and meaning of the kuji-in rituals. You will find the specific details of how Kuji-in works.

These performed are not found in the literature

To learn ninjutsu you must also rely heavily on a limited number of other people.

Sources not directly linked to the historical shinobi

arts.

Hayes (Lepine) states that each of the 9 are distinct.

Kuji have a special philosophy associated with them

A master of competence will teach the student.

You can then consider what to do after you have completed the assigned task.

Hand-seal and mantra (mudra).49-50 The kuji are to remain

In a systematic manner, you will progress through each step.

The philosophical contemplation, mastery and wisdom of Rin.51Each

Kuji named Rin is based on the philosophies.

The ramifications for the previous seals--one does not skimp

The practice can be found all around. This is a brief and eclectic summary of

Each character's philosophy is the following:

Rin: The practitioner begins to realize that he/she does have the right and develops faith in the universe to guide him/her.

One could also focus on cultivating an unfailing mind and strong spirit to endure difficult situations.54

Kyo: One learns to see and accept the karmic cycle that accompanies one's actions.

Toh: Toh refers to one's ability to develop intuition.60

Sha: The practitioner integrates the philosophical saliencies of the preceding three seals to declare the power and right to channel one's energies for necessitated purposes including the healing of others and oneself.61,62Alternatively the practitioner may cultivate the power of Sha to enhance control of one's body and that of another.63

Kai: This is when the practitioner begins to appreciate and practice a philosophy based on loving compassion for everyone through recognition and appreciation of one's existential roots. 64 He/she also recognizes that all human experience are inexorable manifestations and that the universe experiences itself through the activities and interactions of all things. To this end, it is possible to view difficult situations in life as an invitation to explore the root causes. A person's life has a purpose and value that is determined by the fact their life is immutably integral to the overall structure. A connection to the universal mind may allow one to have supernatural or 'extrasensory' abilities of intuition.65 This ability is believed to aid the shinobi when detecting danger before it happens.66

Jin: A practitioner brings to fruition the ability of speaking and listening to, or inferring the thoughts and intentions, of others.67.68.69 A general willingness to learn new information is also a characteristic. The philosophy and philosophies of Jin are a mixture of the previous seal philosophies.

Retsu (Religious Training): A practitioner should approach all objects and phenomena of life with an innocent and receptive mind. The practitioner is believed over time to be able to access subtle realms that may not otherwise be available to the general public.70,71

Zai: One sees oneself as essentially spiritual and merges with the source. This recognition of the inseparability in one's manifest existence from the universe scheme becomes a source power for realizing the will to spirit.

Zen: To attain enlightenment, one must master this kuji.

Hypnotism

There have been claims that the occult practice of

Nijutsu also included hypnosis.

Functioned as a facilitator in the capture and management of an enemy's thoughts.

However, this idea does not agree with what has already been stated

The 20th-century Japanese historian of ninjutsuGingetsuItoh muddying water the waters. Itoh insists on the fact that historical and modern ninjutsu have no relationship whatsoever with hypnosis.

arts.

As was already done in the opening

statements of the current work, there remain the

Potential for some hidden traditions of ninjutsu

Incorporate "hypnotism". But you should not include documentation.

Any claim of ninja-training and tactics

Hypnosis is not a valid method of communication.

The philosophy that guided the skillful use of shinobi was

It wasn't something that was achieved early in life; rather, it was the result a lifetime of practice.

Matters of Prudential conduct

All of the things a shinobi did were probably possible

well-reasoned. Let's take, for instance, the one rule of conduct.

It was advised that shinobi adhere to the principle of not lying.80

This advice may seem ironic, given the fact that the Shinobi have a similar opinion.

Functioned using deceptive techniques, but upon closer examination

Inspection shows that the real reason is lying.

Avoiding is actually a prudent strategy which holds up to the air.

It is a form of deception. This principle is intended promote deception

Building trust in the shinobi and being honest.

person to the extent that a lie will be told when it is considered appropriate

As fact.

It is said that life's vicissitudes are part of the human experience.

The practitioner of Ninjutsu cannot be shocked

The beauty of life is what we are able to make - it is the key to cultivating an

always calm and clear.

Shinobi Code of Conduct

Below is a brief list of behaviors.

A code of conduct. A majority of these

Fujibayashi delimits behavior in "Seishin", Volume

2 Bansenshukai.83

These are the points you can deduce from the following behavior.

It appears that the historical Ninja was more of an actor than a human being.

functionary for higher philosophical principles than an

Incorrigible criminal, without discipline or assassin sans

conscience.

1. Do not tell lies

2. Do not steal for selfish gain

3. Don't cheat

4. Fear not shameful or disgraceful behavior

5. Do not be greedy

6. Don't act too quickly

7. Do not laugh

8. Don't drink

9. Avoid the temptation of lust

10. Do not allies yourself with unprincipled individuals

11. Cherish the truth

Respect your parents

13.Value the higher principles of 'benevolence','fidelity', and 'righteousness' instead of valuing the pleasures of the human senses

Chapter 7: Warfare Principles And Ninjutsu

Although ninjutsu doesn't have a martial element, students will see that it is a method of fostering flexibility in mind as well as body. First, identify the problem. Then use the infinitely powerful salience of human cognition and create a solution.

If we are able to master ninjutsu, as a method of self-defense, then we can think outside the box of what our feet and hands can do to help us solve our problems. It can teach us to think clearly and to use intelligence to solve problems. This is why studying ninjutsu matters.

Fujibayashi states, "While the methods or techniques of the older shinobi can prove effective and should be highly regarded, it is equally important to understand that there principles that underlie these methods which can be adapted to all circumstances." They can be applied to self-defense techniques by anyone who takes the time to study them.

Shochu Kokoruzuke no Koto for instance, refers to the art of paying more attention to the insects in your environment. Shigenori's words could be read and understood by one person. When one digs deeper, one sees that the art has its foundations in a principle. In this example, it is the principleof situational awareness.

You can apply this principle to a modern environment and pay attention the activity in one's surroundings. This will allow you to discover meaning behind seemingly inconsequential events.

The sudden flight of birds away from a wooded environment is not only a significant event, but can also be interpreted as a warning sign that a possible predator is present. The mind begins to associate objects and activity with different phenomena, which can lead to a depth of awareness about one's environment that isn't possible for most people.

You would be wrong to think that you could still practice true Nijutsu in this day and age. True Ninjutsu was primarily created for war purposes, as we have seen in previous chapters.

Fast-forward to 21st century, and the spy-game is changing dramatically in terms techniques, weapons, and tools. The camera and satellite are now more powerful than the once-silent scout who provided tactical intelligence to enemy troops.

Equipments to acquire battlefield information. Even the spy dressed as a monk on the road has been replaced in the creation deceitful online identities.

Today, the warfare functions performed by the ninja are being replaced by electronic surveillance techniques, information dragnets, special forces, and a range of personnel, services, and personnel of three-letter agents (CIA FBI, NSA and NSA). It would be wrong to add the term "ninjutsu", to any one of these examples. It would imply the true practitioners of ninjutsu were active even in 17th-century Japan when the skills were said to have died out.

No, true Ninjutsu can no longer be practiced. However, its principles and techniques are still alive in the manuals written by Natori Mazumi, Fujibayashi Yasutake Chikamatsu Shigenori, and other members of the Hattori family.

The principle is to be as informed as possible about enemy objective properties.

This principle may be used to make better plans for camping trips in unfamiliar areas. One modern example of this principle is to visit the area before you go and take pictures of the terrain. This will allow you to identify potential predators and water sources. It also allows you to locate other resources and useful facilities. More information is better. The trip plan can then be incorporated from this information. Even though this is a common example, it's not the only one that could be used.

2. Infiltration of Qualitative Information and Analysis/Observation

0 This article refers to infiltrating an interest area prior to fighting. The article differs from its predecessor in that it details what type of information is possible to gather. Instead of focusing on predominantly objective/quantitative information, the historical shinobi may also be used in acquiring information of a subjective/qualitative value. To provide information of an enemy's internal atmosphere (emotions or level of thinking), the shinobi can be returned to the commander. Other troop attributes can be used to gain an advantage. The shinobi can inspect the enemy's training, moral disposition, or capabilities for valor/bravery.

0 Modern Application

Psychological Operations

The espionage aspect of Shinobi-no jutsu can be found here

roots in a careful analysis of Sun Tzu's Art of War.

He continues to be of great service to military tacticians today.

Chikamatsu Shigenori says to his readers, "Iga and..."

Shinobi no-jutsu Shinka Koka traditions put emphasis on

Sun Tzu's work in particular, is worth reading carefully

4

This section of The Art of War focuses on the art of war.

Short, only a handful of pages in the

Translation available to this writer Although admittedly,

This compactness can sometimes be deceiving and make it easy to overlook its inner.

Secrets to remain forever elusive to the person who does not read

You can read between the lines and see the potential applications

Instead of specific techniques, they are principles.

What is of special interest?

Individuals who are interested in investigating the connection between

Shinobi operatives and the modern psychological

Sun Tzu's instruction that "expendables" be used in operations

Spy agents to disseminate false information among

enemy.5

day armies to support psychological operations

Sun Tzu's directive to manipulate

information about the enemy

Psychological Operations Tactics. Techniques. and Procedures

The purpose of a psychological operation is to treat the patient.

(PYSOP), the goal is to "convey certain information and indicator"

to target foreign audiences...to impact their emotions

Motives and objective reasoning are the basis of behavior.

Organizations, governments, and groups from abroad

Individuals."6 This is an even more modern version

Sun Tzu's principle of using expendable spies

It is well-known that propaganda dissemination can be done by media.

A variety of modern psychological operations are available, depending on the

Situations may need to be spread by covert means

Transport agents such as these who are willing to risk their lives.

Distribute these materials."7

Contrary to what "psychological operations" of the time

Period during which most likely shinobi operators were involved

Contemporary PSYOPs are more powerful and effective than ever.

Technological span increased by the emergence unheard of technologies

Technological advances in electronic "mass communication"

Use print type.8

Drops or oration of a selected spy group or spy group

To disseminate propagandism, it is easy to imagine.

Modernized principles would apply to shinobi.no-jutsu.

Colored using particular techniques, which include leaflet

Drops from radio/cable/internet broadcasts, airplanes

Different media are used for message distribution. Respective single agents participating in a massive

PSYOP, a modern technique for spreading information

For military purposes, the use of

Apparel, mannerisms and linguistic colloquialisms are all part of the "Manetisms" category.

To gain rapport with a target group for manipulation through, one should display a basic image of a "commonman", or a person who reflects this image.

This information can be derived by ancient ninjutsu texts. Fujibayashi, in his Bansenshukai, points out the importance of learning the language, dress, and customs of the people from each region.

The Shinobi hiden encourages this12 and Chikamatsu Chigenori expounds on a Koka Nija tradition that requires a shinobi understand the "character of a people"13. This includes the effective dissemination of propaganda and casual intelligence-gathering activities. Antonio J. Mendez a former CIA operative, discusses in The Master of Disguise how he used Buddhist beliefs to benefit from one particular propaganda campaign. This is evidently impossible without an in-depth understanding of the culture and beliefs that target populations hold.

Guerilla Warfare and Incendiary Disciplines

Modern texts about guerilla fighting have parallels

The guerilla tactics of shinobi in particular the use

Incendiary devices It is well-known for example that

Shinobi were used by the enemy to break into fortifications.

They were set ablaze. This tactic helped to split the enemy

As many men as necessary to mobilize forces

The fires. The confusion continued as the other enemy soldiers surrounded them.

they would be engaged by a strike of shinobi allies

team.

The U.S. Army Special Forces Guide on Unconventional

Warfare contains incendiary recipes and techniques

Devices for sabotage wooden structures

as well other combustible victims. This is evidence that the principle underpinning the shinobi Saboteur is still in use within modern armies.

Cameras & Counter-Surveillance

Technology has given criminals new ways to approach victims in modern society. To be able to defend oneself, it is essential that you become aware of your vulnerabilities.

Surveillance techniques can take many unexpected forms that give the user a significant advantage over the targeted target. These technologies are likely simple with respect to their components. They typically consist of a microphone paired with a camera. Surveillance systems are simple to disguise as other innocuous, mundane items.

Fig. 5.1) are two images of a computer bag modified to conceal a camera that was discreetly mounted into one side panel. The camera inside the bag can be connected to its battery supply and a portable recording unit for digital video (DVR).

Anyone can buy or create a similar system, and then place it within the immediate vicinity of a target to gather information without suspicion.

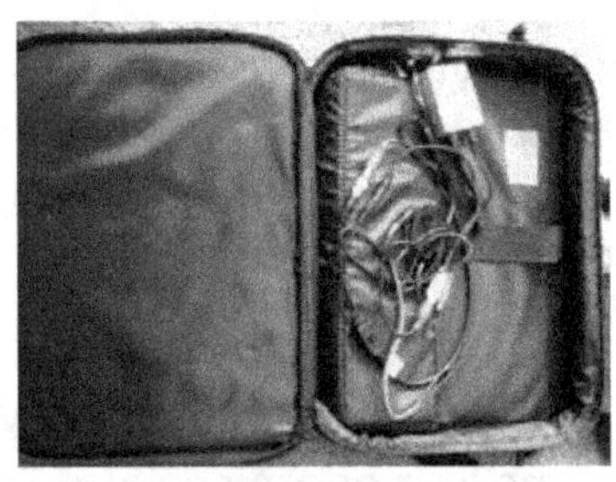

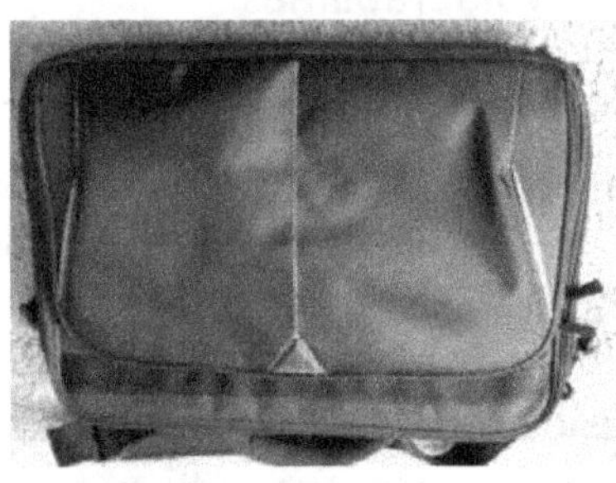

(fig. 4.1)

A hidden camera's disguise can be any number of things. For example, it can appear as a tree, pen, coffee cup, or even an electrical outlet. As surveillance systems are not always predictable, it would be better for potential victims to become more aware of the possibility that they could be under covert surveillance at any moment.

This awareness must be combined with the determination to disregard surveillance systems and display unpredictable behavior. This includes breaking patterns of behavior, leaving home at random times and even setting up countersurveillance (deploy a system to monitor for suspicious activity). Whatever your choice, the key point is to know what the enemy's tricks and techniques are. This will enable you to devise effective counter-measures for those who would maliciously employ them.

How could someone use surveillance technology to achieve malicious ends?

In general surveillance is used to gather intelligence about the intended target. This information can then be used to guide future tactical decisions. When protecting yourself against surveillance, it is important not to forget that adequate surveillance prior an assault or an attack is a patient procedure that does NOT owe any allegiance whatsoever to any side.

Public debate has been focused on terrorism as ISIS has received recruits from the U.S. Some believe that there could be an attack anywhere in the world any minute now. In an effort to deter terroristic activities, the Boston Police Department issued a "brochure" listing certain surveillance behaviors.

1. Initiating a deliberate act that results in a response from law enforcers to make it easy for them to "response" times.

2. Video and photography are used to capture specific locations and events.

3. The area is mapped.

Terrorists, as shown above, use the same kinds of warfare principles and tactics as the shinobis of history. By studying ninjutsu one can develop a counter to terroristic activities in that potential victims of terroristic actions are educated (know the enemy) to some extent.

Security as a corrupted nature

As a watchman or guard, your job is simple. You just need to observe the surroundings and report anything amiss.

Being a good security guard requires a lot of observation and memory. One might lose your way by stealing, breaking into, or manipulating employees to gain access to the things they desire. This is why it is important to remember that manipulation of the security guard's or watchman's function, especially that of observation can lead to malicious or deviant ends.

Tendo Chido Narai refers to a Shoninki chapter that offers insight into this possibility.15 Natori also explains in it, that shinobi should be skilled at swaying the sensemediated observation of sentinels up toward the sky or down low depending on the target.

Let's say that someone wanted to get into a very secure area through a tunnel. The tunnel is often guarded only by foot patrols. To ensure the plan to enter in this way, the infiltrator might display a strange display (e.g., fireworks, holographic projectionors, fleets of Chinese floating lanterns, etc.). The infiltrator may place lights in the sky to draw attention to the guards and direct them away from entry points. Only the most seasoned sentinel or knowledgeable would question if such a ploy was really intended to distract potential gaps in security perimeter.

Similar to the above scenario, if one wants to enter from above (say a roof), the clever infiltrator will use a distraction below. There are many tricks that can be used to cover up a particular situation. An accomplice could fake a heart attack and sudden onset illness. A doorman might also be rude and argue with him to make a scene. The intruder would have the option of entering the facility through a roof-bound window while security is distracted.

Social engineers with innate skills and common criminals may use the principle that swaying attention to heavens or earth might be employed by gifted social workers. Security guards and watchmen should have the ability to identify their own weaknesses. It is incredible to see how security functions can make an area more insecure.

Chapter 8: Incorporating Ninjutsu Principles For

Selfdefense

"Self-defense" is a term that refers to protective actions taken in order to resist a physical attack. It is most often used by martial artists. They may alter a traditional art's technique in a way that makes it compatible with current assault/battery techniques. It can be said that all arts offer some form useful training to students interested to'self-defense'. However, this is only true if the term is used to refer to the physical attack of the fists/kicks variety (sometimes as weapons).

To be clear, selfdefense is not limited to hand-to-hand combat. It should include a broad concept that protects oneself against almost any type of harm or attack. True self-defense could be described as a way that one lives, which minimizes dangers and stresses the importance of maintaining a level of defense against crime and violence.

One can understandably assume that if one is not prepared for every situation, then one will be weak everywhere. Take this into consideration: all methods of self defense are based upon easily absorbed, adaptable principles. It is possible to learn the principle and be more equipped to provide a defense that addresses your specific issue.

"Principles, not Techniques"

Let's take a look at Bansenshukai. We will see if the principles found therein are complementary or alternative to modern ideas on warfare and self defense.

Did the ninja, aka the shinobi possess skills with the foot, fist, and hand? It's obvious they did.

Is there a shinobi-only style of hand-to-hand combat? This is where things get complicated.

These questions will be addressed in the future, but here are some key points to remember:

1. Shinobi no jutsu, an adjunct art, was a form of fighting that was taught to samurai. These samurai were usually already skilled in hand-tohand combat skills. Logic would suggest that a fighting method for a ninja was based on samurai combatives, and that it could vary from one clan or another.

2. The Shinobi-no jutsu texts such as the Shoninki, Chikamatsu Shigenori's scrolls and the Gunpo Jiyoshu do not contain any hint of hand to hand fighting techniques.

3. For ninjutsu, historical documentation is necessary in order to verify its credibility. Ninja are warriors from the past.

A chronological period that has been forgotten by time. History can only be studied if we rely on texts, relics, or both.

Other archaeological evidence. They cannot resort only to the mere word of alleged "masters". We now exist in the 21st Century, not feudal Japan. It is therefore necessary to have access to archaeologists, historians, and archaeologists for verification of the authenticity a ninjutsu.

I am not an historian by training or profession. I am simply a commoner who has taken time to research historical texts on the subject of ninjutsu, in order to draw conclusions about this attractive but misunderstood arts. However, I must also disclose that I was once a To-Shin Do student (3 years) and that this has allowed me to have an insider's view of the art. It has led me to the unpalatable conclusion that true Ninjutsu is not reflected in any other TSD Dojos.

This journey of finding truth about matters of ninjutsu has taken 8 years. It was sometimes hard work, as I try to make progress towards clarity. Ninjutsu holds a special place in my heart. However, I will not misuse it by pretending to not be aware of the texts (i.e. exalting "ninjutsu" Dojos. These translated texts prove that true ninjas have long since departed this realm. They are only vestiges of their past traditions.

You will see that I don't speak Japanese. I think I am deluded into believing that I can comprehend the art. This is a fine criticism. But I do have to ask who really understands the art. You can point him/her out.

Do we define art by particulars in language, or should we not be so ignorant as to assume principles are defined only by native languages?

The heart of ninjutsu resides in the principles. The principles are the foundation of ninjutsu. You can understand these principles and the value of ninjutsu to self-defense. These principles can easily be inferred and deduced using the texts, which were translated by Yoshie Miami from Antony Cummins's research.

So where does that leave us in regards to our question about ninjutsu or self-defense? I will discuss some of the key principles.

1. It is important to understand the impact information has on your decisions. Shinobi of old were skilled in spreading propaganda to manipulate the psychology. It is essential that we learn to recognize truth in our information-rich society. Because it was often that he was faced

with a situation where he had to cut through the fog, logic was essential for shinobis.

Enemy ninjas spread misinformation. It is important to realize that everything we do contains information of some type. Everything you do, from what you drive to how you dress to the content of your social media pages to your online traffic and even your choice of flags for your yard, can reveal a lot about your personality and inner psychology. What are your enemies' perceptions of you, if they exist?

2. Be prepared for difficult times. You must be prepared to face difficult situations. Shinobi for instance were known to have a lot of bushcraft skills that allowed them to be able to survive in the face of danger (this is "self-defense"). This doesn't mean you have to go out and learn how the land works, although that can be helpful. But it does mean you need an assessment of your existence (e.g. The location of your home, demographics, criminal record, access to utilities, and personal characteristics all matter. To protect yourself from the pain that could result from the breakdown of any systems you rely upon.

3. Be able to think outside the boxes of traditional defense methods. It is easy, however, to be drawn into the currents that promote selfdefense sensationalism. This profits the peddlers weapons, a macho mentality or extreme strength.

Rarely do we consider that the greatest soldier is not one who has to fight. Similar to medicine, in which the superior doctor is someone who prevents a disease instead of treating it, so the superior warrior is proactive in eliminating the root causes of conflict, rather than engaging in violently in its blossoming. There's more glory in avoiding danger and war than in winning over it.

"Those who are skilled in shinobi arts can have no enemies." Natori Sanjuro Masazumi

4. Know what you are willing or unable to give up. The shinobi pledged allegiance and loyalty to his lord until his death. To whom do you need to answer? Your family? Your family members? Do you want to go as far as possible in defense of yourself or the ones you love?

Goshiki Mai (5-colored rice)

This ancient ninjutsu practice involves the deposition or placement of colored rice within an operation area in order to send information to allies. The shinobi would use various colors to color the rice. He/she would carry bamboo tubes with him/her. To avoid decryption attempts, the rice would be stored in accordance with a predetermined, closely guarded code-key. Different color rice arrangement could have different meanings. Only those with the key can decode the message.

Method Incontinences: 1. Possible disturbance of the coded messaging by animals, climactic and human interaction 2. Communication distance and accuracy of reception (recipient must stay within 20 feet minimum of rice in order for the message to be decoded) 3. The potential to raise suspicion (Why does there appear to be colored rice?

Method Advantages

Use: This method works well when the weather does not forecast to bring heavy rain or wind (rain, snow, and so on). Your messages should be left in plain sight, but clearly visible. It may help you to inform.

Communication team about which method of placement is preferable (i.e. By trees or on rocks, alongside roads, etc. You shouldn't have to carry a lot of colored rice. The amount you use for each message should also be limited. It is important to create a crypto-key and rice placement patterns. Each member of the communications team should be trained on the type information that will be transmitted (this will vary depending upon the situation). Team members should be informed about protocol in case a coded communication appears to have been altered. Make sure that senders practice message redundancy. Place the same code twice, in two different areas. Guard the cryptkey.

Escape and Evasion with Lockpicking

Stephen Nojiri has documented it well, as Antony Cummins. It is known that lockpicking is part of the skillsets of a shinobi.

This art could have been used for various purposes, such as escaping capture or sneaking into restricted areas. You can apply this principle by learning the components and security features of modern locks. You could start by buying a lockpick set or creating your own tools with flexible, durable metals. To practice pragmatically, you can purchase several tumbler lock pins.

Moku Ton-Jutsu & CCW w/ a Hoodie - Modernized Shinobi-no-jutsu Strategies

Don' t undervalue your common hoodie. You won't believe it, but this fabric is full and ready for use.

The concealed carry permit holders who own a hoodie may use it as a concealment or retention holster. Depending on the colour of the clothing and the bulk of the material, this technique provides comparable concealment performance to standard holsters. However, I wouldn't carry a gun that way if a better holster was readily available.

It is important to practice drawing with concealment weapons. The gun may snag. It's possible to wear too thin material, which will make it difficult for you to see the profile of your tool. This article serves only informational purposes and I am not responsible to your inability or unwillingness to train safely. You may also need a CCW permit to do so. The following describes a technique for drawing a hoodie:

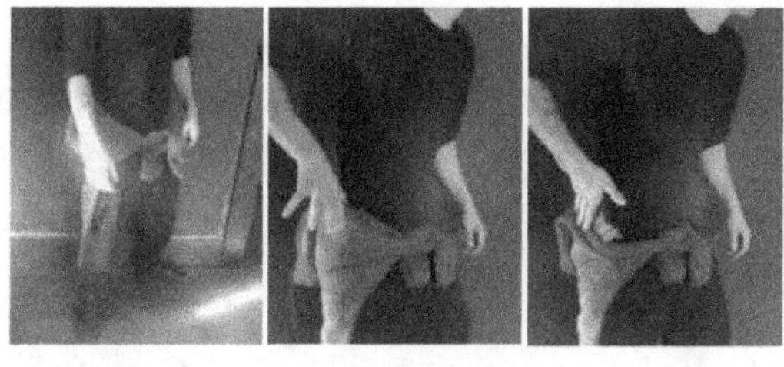

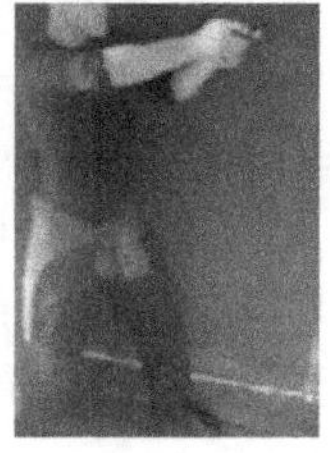

The color scheme used herein isn't important. However, I will state that a darker color hoodie allows a lower tool profile. Your thumb will guide the firearm to its open display (photo 2). Then, grip and draw. Once again, practice...practice...practice. Anyone who wishes learn this method should practice it by carrying an empty firearm around the home. This is to help build confidence and comfort with the technique so that one is able to know how to properly holster the firearm. If the technique is worthwhile, additional magazine holders and a muzzle-holder can be added to your jacket depending on your life circumstances. Be creative, but realistic. Hoodies are a popular article of clothing. However, you should think about how they can be useful beyond protecting your skin from the elements.

Gingestu Itoh, a researcher in ninjutsu of the 20th century, defined moku ton-jutsu at "techniques which involve evading, fleeing or otherwise, concealing your body within trees and grasses."4 I have not been able to find any historically documented cases in which shinobi used trees to escape capture. But it is evident that the shinobi were skilled at hiding themselves within the foliage of the forest.

Shinobis are believed to have used their obi belts to climb trees. A shinobi would not use his obi belt for climbing trees. One can instead use a jacket as a climbing tool to reach those difficult trees without branches. It's simple enough. You might feel like you are a lumber-jack. I know it felt that way. Do not forget to wrap your hands in the loose ends of the Hoodie.

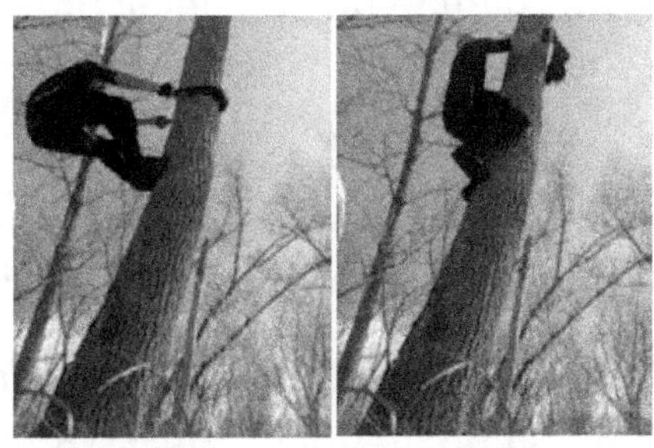

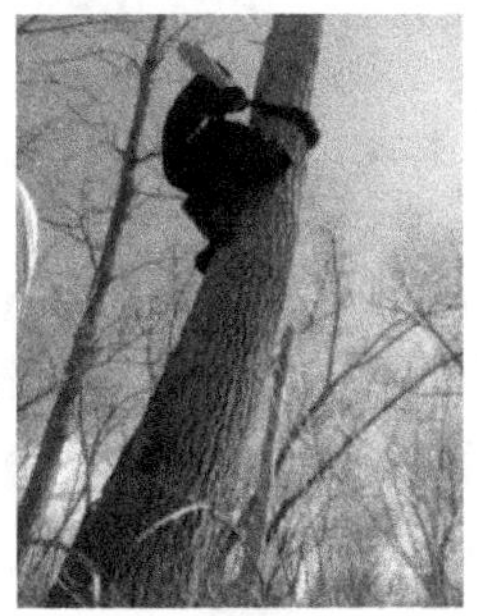

Appendix 1: Shadow Zone Material

This section contains articles on Ninjutsu you can find on Shadow Zone (www.shadowzone.net).

Ninjutsu is a Creative Process

"If we had to examine one meaning of Ninjutsu, it would be that the term is purely...a set enduring techniques." Gingetsu Itoh

How can a thing be defined? It's like asking "What is Nijutsu?" What are the steps to define it?

Since symbols are used for describing phenomena, ninjutsu defies observation as its phenomena are contained to the past. Naturally, we cannot explain, let alone delineate, what is not visible.

When defining ninjutsu for the first time, we have to rely heavily on cultural and social conventions as well a few historical records. Many of these records are similar to modern intelligence agencies. The possibility that "kuden", which would clarify our knowledge of ninjutsu, might haunt us means that our understanding will be limited. The conclusion is that the true boundaries and boundaries of the art won't be known to us. We only have a small amount shinobi knowledge.

We don't stress about it, but we do not worry. Instead, our enthusiasm is infectious as we dive into the records. Language barriers become another obstacle in our quest for defining ninjutsu.

Similar to the English language and many other modifications have been made throughout the centuries to the Japanese Language. Without a modern expert in the historical ninjutsu language, we will invariably be searching for the essence. (And even if we have a translator, we may not know all).

Summarizing: We have a diluted vestige of ninjutsu which we can keep. This is why I feel compelled to explore the concepts of the arts and make something new from themashes. If we want to keep ninjutsu's "heart" alive, we need to apply its principles to the contemporary world.

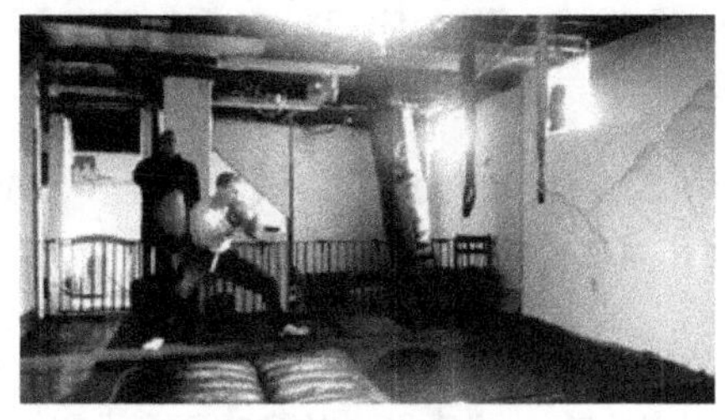

Basic Scouting, and Emergency Planning: Knowing the Territory

Scouting is a lesser-known aspect of ninjutsu.

You should know that "ninjutsu", modern dojos, which focus on rumination on martial arts techniques instead of the rudimentary functions a shinobi leader can't be trusted to teach their students the most practical of ancient ways of shinobi that could save them in times when they are in dire need. The history of ninjutsu teaches us that observation, which is the ability to perceive, appraise, and record information, was an essential part of the art. If you're not learning to see a target and conduct basic surveillance, or even survey an entire territory (and what purpose), you're missing a vital step on your way.

This post will focus on the value of Ninjutsu, as it applies to planning for emergencies. Before I go on, we need to look at the history of ninjutsu. It was practiced during feudal periods.

Here are some questions for you to get us started.

* Why did Shinobi scout territory (i.e. What was its purpose and context?

* How did shinobi find a territory? (i.e. What equipment were used and what methodologies?

* Are the principles of ninjutsu scouting/surveillance still applicable today?

It is well-known to everyone that shinobi are often used as spies. Scroll after scroll can be found historical references which state that the function a ninja had was to 'know the enemy'. This fulfills Sun Tzu's advice to commanders that they must know the capabilities of the armies of their troops. According to Art of War shinobi can provide essential intelligence to any army.

Shinobi traveled to territories to find intelligence that could help their lords if there was ever a crisis. They assessed the infrastructure, roads as well as ports, watercourses, and the behavioral dispositions of the residents of the region. The number of relevant regional detail categories that these agents discovered were sufficient to allow Yo-nin penetration of the community in question should their commander issue a directive.

As tempting as it is to consider the shinobi an individual "master" who can will and control all of his forces, we must also understand that his services were part in a well-organized feudal army machine. This meant that his skills were only available if an order from a higher authority was given. Contrary, the idea of shinobi self-reliance has been disproven by such ninjutsu texts and the Bansenshukai proving that an agent's loyalty to higher authority was a critical determinant in the success or failure of a mission.

Summa sum, the "why" behind shinobi-scouting revolved about military success, and thus the survival or the domain of his ruler. Insomuch that modern students of ninjutsu do not have "lords", the corollary arises that the truest application of ninjutsu's surveillance/scouting functions is a thing of the past. The skills of scouting, despite their declining military status in the Edo period, are still valid and used by the shinobi.

This brings us to our next question, "How did Shinobi Scout?"

There are many options for methods that a Shinobi might use, depending on the circumstance. Some of these are covered within the Hoi no Maki ("Volume of Principles") of Chikamatsu Shigenori. Agents are advised to travel extensively, visit as many towns or territories as possible, to get valuable contacts or informants, as well as to learn the area's customs and dress codes, as well as the dispositions of military personnel and more.

This information was obtained through human interaction and the use of their senses. It was possible to record this information by either recording it to long-term storage or by making detailed notes with a seihetsu ("stone pencil") to keep track of the details. Some cleverer ways to record information were also invented. Shinobi could count items or people of particular interest by dropping beans onto the ground. After completing his count, he would subtract from the total the beans he had in his pocket the number he began with to determine the value. This method could be used to count large numbers, without him attracting attention.

Ninjutsu Scouting can be used to help with emergency preparedness

While we do have no feudal lords we can still improve our security and response capabilities to crisis situations by applying the intelligence gathering functions that ninjutsu offers to the modern day. Instead of gathering intelligence on enemy capability, we can gather intelligence in the surroundings and outlying areas that will help us to plan for our emergency response. After identifying the most likely crises or calamities to hit your country, you can begin to apply ninjutsu into your emergency preparedness strategy by doing these:

* Get familiar with the local maps. Pay attention to waterways, population centres, distances between communities, the size and layout of each municipality, city, and country.

* Save detailed photographs of maps to you phone and retain physical copies.

* Calculate distances between points. two cities, your nearest water-source, etc. You can travel by foot or in a car.

* Explore the roads. Buy an onboard camera to help you monitor your vehicle's movements and record important information.

* You will need to remember the county codes in order to locate plates within your area.

* Go to the closest town or city in your locality. Visit them every now and again, and gradually increase your awareness to other places.

* If you are visiting other locations, make sure to be aware of the infrastructure (bridges/tracks/waterways, buildings, railway tracks, waterways), emergency services such as hospitals, police stations and fire stations, FEMA points, etc. It is important to know the areas' industries (types of employment) and the potential camping spots. Mix with locals at gathering places such as churches, general stores, or restaurants to learn more about the surroundings.

* Prepare for an emergency evacuation by noting which localities are possible to store supplies. Because caches can be hidden in forested areas

or foliated terrain, I prefer recreational spots for this purpose.

* Learn how supplies caches can withstand all the elements. These caches contain life-sustaining equipment such a firestarter, ammunition, food, water, cordage and medical supplies.

* Form a network with shadow preppers. Establish a network of shadow preppers if you have made contact with someone in a distant location.

You can communicate with him.

Intelligence Gathering: Fundamentals

Because shinobi were originally spies, it's reasonable to expect that anyone who attempts to recreate, discuss, and practice ninjutsu to do so in accordance with the verifiable truth, is also to possess knowledge of "the art or intelligence" today.

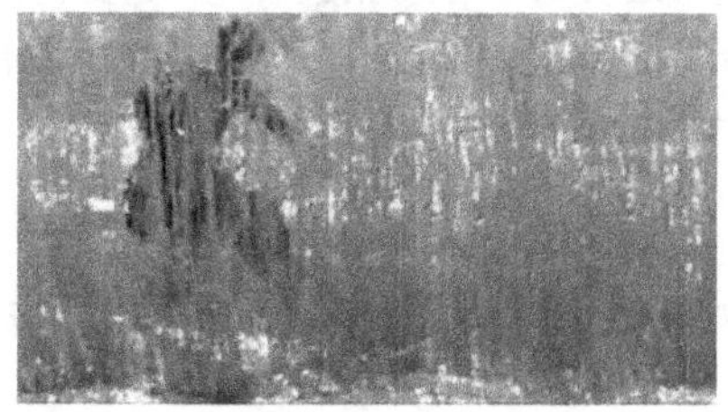

The art of intelligence has deep roots. Espionage is considered the most important element of any successful military operation. This art has been adopted by many cultures, and it remains essential to military affairs. It is possible to surmise that spying was used in order to keep power or to aid in the removal of perceived enemies. Imagine the activities of these pro-spies, who skulked around to obtain vital information from conversations.

Unfortunately, imagination is not enough to bring to life a large number of spymen who will never be discovered by humankind... because they were involved in the trade and distribution of secrets. Similar with the shinobi. We will never know exactly how many there were or how their lives were.

They developed their methods of gathering intelligence using limited technology and their human senses in the distant future. Shinobi had no cameras or satellites like 21st-century spy, so their methods of intelligence gathering were limited to creativity, the human sensorium, and not satellites.

Shinobi needed to have sharp eyes and a great memory to be successful. The information that was recorded would then be transmitted to the relevant party. Human senses can be trained. Shinobi may have had their own methods of sharpening these skills. What we really need to know about espionage is the ability to use your senses and have a good memory in order acquire specific information.

How much information did the shinobi have? Anything that could have revealed the dispositions of the target could have been very valuable. The Yokan Denkai is focused on the retrieval of details about the political and justice systems of the enemy. There is much more information that ninjutsu can provide.

Let me stop there and emphasize another component of intelligence gathering: Secretiveness is implicit to the practice or gaining information on an enemy.

If a spy doesn't know how deceive his enemy, he won't live long after he has been discovered. Human creativity is key here. This intelligence principle, which is secretive and deceitful, guides all aspects of ninjutsu.

Understanding this we see that the core of ninjutsu is the principle secretion in gathering intelligence. Ninjutsu seems also to have developed around this principle.

The same principles inherent to ninjutsu may also be found within modern intelligence modalities. Thanks to their timeless nature and adaptability, we can still make use of them in our everyday lives with a little imagination.

Why should we include intelligence in our own self-protection system or preparedness skillsetset? Sun Tzu stated that to defeat the enemy we must know ourselves and understand the enemy. Self-assessment and introspection can help us meet the first condition. Only when we are able to understand and practice intelligence can the second condition be fulfilled.

But there is one caveat. Don't allow yourself to be blinded by the temptation to see your enemy only through your eyes. It is important that your strategy sees you through the enemy's eyes. Without your knowledge, he might be looking at you. This is a great way to see how everything you publish about yourself can be used against, especially if your enemy is skilled in this area. This is the case with social engineers. If you don't know what they are, I recommend you search for them online.

Sensory Training Candle Meditation

Place a small candle at a distance from where your intention to sit. Turn off the lights and light the candle. Then, relax into a comfortable meditation position. Pay attention to the flame. Pay attention its size, colors, movements, and movements. Relax your breathing. Take a mental photo of the candle at varying times and then return to the stare. Continue this process for as many times as you want.

An Introduction to Innin

Fujibayashi thinks In-nin, pronounced eeeen, skills are less important than Yonin (Open Disguise), infiltration skills. However the former has been what made the ninjas popular.

In-jutsu involves a shinobi climbing a castle wall or hiding among trees to assess the target. Injutsu has the dark garb of the shinobi, the breaking and entering of tools, and the secretive movement strategies of the ninja. Yojutsu involves deceiving your enemy using clever use of disguises, speech, behavior, and other tactics.

Fujibayashi advises us not to forget that In-jutsu doesn't work well without Yo-jutsu. Hence, both arts must be studied.

Defining In-jutsu

In-jutsu describes techniques for hiding from or stealing someone into a target of interests using camouflage techniques, tools, and hiding methods (Ongyo.no.jutsu). The

Bansenshukai offers us examples of Innin through 'Dojun", who invaded Sawayama castle, first disguised himself as "lumberjack", a Yoo-nin skill.

Dojun is said that he switched to Injutsu once he had gotten in the way of Yo-nin.

Another example is Suyama/Komiyama's In-nin Infiltration Methods. This story was told by Komiyama under heavy rainstorm. Komiyama used grapplinghooks to infiltrate Kasagi temple defenses.

Suyama Yoshitaka was the leader of Hojo forces in the Genko War's "Siege of Kasagi", 1331-1333. KomiyamaJiro was stationed within the fortified Kasagiyama temple. The siege ended only after Komiyama (Suyama) quietly scaled Kasagiyama's rock faces with grapplinghooks. They did this at night under the cover of a storm. After climbing the mountain, the enemy stopped them and asked them questions. Suyama (and Komiyama) are said to have fooled troops by pretending that they were Go'daigo's own men. Komiyama replied that they were part of a night-patrol to catch shinobi. The deception was accepted by the troops who then let them go. As they advanced towards their target the agents would encounter more troops. They would tell them to be vigilant against infiltrators by shinobi every time they saw more troops. Once they had found and rescued the emperor from the temple fortress's walls, they set the temple ablaze. Shinobi arson is at its best.

Practice skills in realistic situations is the best way for you to transfer your knowledge to a real-world situation. You won't be able to prepare for an enemy that reacts, responds or attacks in the same way you did in your dojo.

This principle can be applied to training in any subject. To master fire-extinguisher use, you need to be able to smell and feel the smoke as you put the fire out. The training wheels need to be removed if you want a good ride on a bike. To parachute you must jump from the plane.

The reality of learning ninjutsu requires a different level of reality than can be found at a dojo.

But what about if?

What if you had the means to learn all the sub-disciplines in ninjutsu. What would be illegal? And what could you pretend to be law-abiding?

The Legal Implications of Ninjutsu Training: A Few Examples

To start, we must define which aspects we want to evaluate in order to determine their function in modern society. Because we don't reside in feudal Japan, certain traditions of adjuncts to ninjutsu must also be discarded.

It is possible to use ninjutsu to help us in our current time. In reality, you won't find yourself requiring you to learn Japanese, but you may need to pick up a lock or fake illness. Watch some videos, peruse the text, and chat with your teacher. List down all the ninjutsu skill you'd like to learn. After that, you might begin to determine what you can legally learn and what would not be legal.

Today I'm going to focus on my favourite ninjutsu subjects: lockpicking, shadow surveillance (following target), taijutsu/body movement/ techniques), lockpicking, and kajutsu.

Lockpicking is a legal skill that can be learned. You will need to purchase or make the equipment required (i.e. picks, boltcutters, tensioners, locks, etc.) Make sure you have somewhere to place the locks so you can mimic a real-world situation. You can choose to have a friend assist you with infiltrating the room that has a lock. Once you start to pick locks that you don't own, the legal boundary blurs. I started lock-picking with a pair Smith and Wesson handcuffs and some cheap padlocks.

Locksmithing in general can be a very complex field that requires a lot more research and effort than you might think.

Taijutsu - This can be any technique the body uses to perform with agility or finesse. I love running up walls and climbing on to buildings. Taijutsu has a lot of legality and will likely make up the majority in modern ninjutsu. Taijutsu training is possible by attending a taijutsu dojo. I have been able to learn back-flips as well as wall-runs by using trees. You must attend a Dojo if you want to learn how you can break someone's neck.

Shadow surveillance: If you are caught stalking someone, you could face serious consequences. Unfortunately, this is how you get better at foot surveillance if you don't have someone to help you.

Ka-jutsu, for the most parts, is illegal to learn. The US BATFE, Bureau of Alcohol Tabacco Firearms and Explosives, enforces laws against the manufacture of explosives, fireworks and incendiaries. You will not be able to use the licence. Any of the above is extremely illegal. Therefore, realistic training is impossible (why would anyone want to torch down a village). You can find legal shinobi designs in ninjutsu handbooks.

I hope you are now able to consider the reasons why modern "ninjutsu" donjos lack so many important elements.

Hideyoshi and the Sword Ban of Hideyoshi, and How the Koka SHinobi Responded

1588, Toyotomi Hiteyoshi, the powerful Toyotomi Hideyoshi, decreed to Japan the "sword hunters" edict.

The common people are being requisitioned for swords, armor, and other items. Hideyoshi used religious references to encourage them to participate in the long peace process to Japan. He also announced that the metal from confiscated swords would go to the construction of a Buddha monolithic sculpture. It was implied that commoners could be freed of some negative karma if they followed the order. This successful campaign to disarm Japan's population led to a clear distinction being made between the nobility versus the peasantry. Samurai can carry the sword; farmers and the less fortunate cannot.

It was a period marked by great change. It was a time for great transition.

Ignorance and darkness are my companions.

Kiumura Okunosuke Yasutaka the sensei from the Koka Ryu traditions, shared his predictions on the fates his ninjutsu Chikamatsu Chigenori. These predictions were recorded by the Koka Shinobi no Den Miraiki (1719 AD).

Kimura says that the younger generation should be included in this document.

Generations whose lineage was tied to the Koka were allowed to relax by the peace of Edo and enjoy a better life. Therefore, the number of those who practice ninjutsu is expected to continue to decline. In the absence of war, peace was making people softened and complacent.

Kimura's story doesn't end here. He speaks of the screening process used to give the Koka Ninjutsu secrets and traditions to the students. He also mentions how only a few people who managed the schools during his time knew a lot about ninjutsu. He explains the necessity of ninjutsu to combat war, and thus he argues for the preservation of the art.

This sensei of Chikamatsu & Koka Ninja

Shigenori responded to Edo's peace by keeping the secrets of the shinobi alive for future generations. Peace can't last forever. For this reason, dark weapons of war should be kept in the attic instead of being burned to the pile.

Modern Reflections about Ninjutsu

Modern 'ninjutsu' dojos often reflect a vivid reanimation, though sometimes quite dilute, of Japanese history. This claim isn't based on an academic acumen steeped into the history of

Japan. It is more an observation that perceives all history and historical imitations as doubtful.

No photographs, videos or audio recordings were available back then to give us an accurate representation of life during the era of the ninjas. We may find their tools, clothing and other artifacts. However, we are left with very little instruction about how they were used. Even though we may have read their texts and can sometimes understand what they were thinking, no translation of Eastern texts can accurately capture the mind of the writer. Language is also a limited conduit to real life. Although experts in history can give some insight to the nature ninjutsu's history, they were not there during that time and so are stuck in the same game of inferring and deducing history.

Do we need to be able to understand ninjutsu correctly? Yes. We can make plausible claims, supported by historical references and texts, that a "ninja" was, did, or was such and such. But we have to remain skeptical. This being said, I'll tell you that I respect ninjutsu and am a pragmatist. I do not want to take anything from the "correct knowledge" of ninjutsu and apply it to my world. I live in a 21st century world with internet, thugs with hand-cannons that rape about with combustionengines and an entirely different legal system which determines what I may or cannot do when attempting to inflict physical violence against an assailant. I can't use a sword to take down someone, or run a clandestine information network (though it would be interesting), and I also cannot carry IEDs in my pocket for my province. I am not Japanese. What benefit can I get from ninjutsu if it is anything that is practical?

Answer: Principles

Principles create specifics. The principles can be used to create real techniques for particular situations. Principles allow the user the freedom to devise his/her own solutions to the fundamental and surreal human threats that the shinobi had to confront (e.g. Flagrant war, death by the sword, covert operations in deceit, or the act of committing suicide at the hands another person. By learning that shinobi were adept in exploiting human and structural weaknesses in order to bypass security we can increase our security awareness regarding contemporary flaws of human sentinel security and physical security. RFID card readers could be one example. You can now 'clone an employee ID card' and trick the RFID reader to gain unauthorized entry to secure areas. As it was his job to infiltrate, a Shinobi would not hesitate to discover such information.

My website, text, and in-person teachings of real ninjutsu are not proof that I teach it. I claim the right of being informed by the nature, principles and practice of ninjutsu. Here are some things I'm relatively certain about in regards to ninjutsu.

1. Ninjutsu had a cerebral aspect. It was less about how proficient you were at using a weapon than it was about how quick you could think on the feet.

2. Referring to Bansenshukai, ninjutsu's essence may be found at 'Seishin', which is the correct mind adviced by Fujibayashi. This is what distinguishes a good ninja from an evil criminal.

3. The above mentioned correctness of thinking reveals the existence of an indomitable spirit within the shinobi. Admiration is due to the ability to persevere through difficult trials, and to maintain correctness of thought.

In my daily life, I don't wear any gi and move around in a Dojo as if it were 15th century knowledge. Recognizing the differences between my past and present, I adopt, emulate, and apply only those principles and precepts of Ninjutsu that still have relevance to today's world. Does that make me a "ninja"? It all depends who you ask.

What if Fujibayashi Shigenori or Natori Maazumi were alive today. How might they determine the character of an person and make it a shinobi-like figure? This is perhaps the question of significance.

The shinobi could do this, without doubt:

Hierarchy. Find out who has power over which areas. He would likely be interested in big business, the government at large, and civil governance down to the lowest level. Why? Because a Shinobi would join hands with a power magnate or lord who might best serve his ideals, family, and community than those that would harm and denigrate everyone else. Confucianism was huge in Japan and China during medieval times. A collectivist mindset, such as what "benefits all the masses," drove the shinobi's decisions. He was loyal in his loyalty to those who promised him order and justice.

Martial Skills. Get comfortable with modern combat, weaponry and tactics. He will likely become immersed in the new "teppo", characterized with machine guns, long distance snipers, and other weapons. The shinobi may also study intelligence according to three letter agencies: the CIA FBI and NSA. Even basic information agents (also known as shinobi) will not hesitate to use the internet and other document repositories in order to gain valuable insights. Sengoku's battles were often fought with heavy armor-wielding warriors. Thus, certain hand/to-hand techniques were necessary to accommodate this situation. The 21st century shinobi will likely have a hand system that is based upon modern realities and attire. He might be interested in MMA or PPCT -Pressure Point Control Tactics - or any other form of physical defense.

Law: Make sure you are familiar with codes and statutes. The Bansenshukai reveals that the Shinobi were part of the arresting of criminals. He was de facto a law enforcement officer and bounty hunter. He was knowledgeable about tactics to deal with criminals locked up in a building and other methods for binding (restraining) the wanted. It is possible that a shinobi could have had a basic understanding about the law.

Cultural surveillance: Watch out for and copy the culture. You can find references after references about how the shinobi was advised that he study the province where he would work. He would need to be familiar with the local dialect and colloquialisms. Additionally, his manners, subject matter, and attire would all match or differ from those who live in the vicinity. He was adept at hiding his identity by mixing in.

Territorial Monitoring: Understand the advantages or disadvantages associated with operations within a specific territory. As a scout, the shinobi worked in both war and peacetime. Shinobi Michi Fumiyo not Koto.

General Surveillance. This course covers both conventional tailing and advanced video surveillance techniques. Black-clad figures in silent pursuit of their targets are one of the most fascinating motifs related to the ninja. There are historical references that show that shinobis from the past could follow their targets on foot in broad daylight and at night without suspicion. The 21st Century shinobi would feel compelled then to learn how use a vehicle to tail his targets.

There is so much more. My fingers are getting tired.

I may add to the list in the future - especially if it is worthwhile by some of you.

Conclusion

I hope you found this book useful. It is possible to get more fit and agile by practicing the techniques and building strength and confidence. It just takes dedication and discipline.

If you found this guide useful and valuable, I would appreciate it if it was shared with your friends. Training with someone will help to keep you motivated and make the training experience more fun. Perhaps you could start your Ninja clan.

I wish your success in your studies!

www.ingramcontent.com/pod-product-compliance
Lightning Source LLC
Chambersburg PA
CBHW051107050726
47592CB00002B/711